Happy, Healthy You

You

Your Total Wellness Toolkit For Renewing Body, Soul, and Mind

KJ LANDIS, BS, Ed, CPT, CFT.

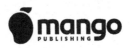

Published by Mango Publishing Group, a division of Mango Media Inc.

Cover Design: Roberto Núñez

Layout & Design: Morgane Leoni

For permission requests, please contact the publisher at:

Mango Publishing Group

2850 Douglas Road, 3rd Floor

Coral Gables, FL 33134 USA

info@mango.bz

For special orders, quantity sales, course adoptions and corporate sales, please email the publisher at sales@mango.bz. For trade and wholesale sales, please contact Ingram Publisher Services at customer.service@ingramcontent.com or +1.800.509.4887.

Library of Congress Cataloging-in-Publication number: 2017907498

Name: KJ Landis

Happy, Healthy You: Your Total Wellness Toolkit for Renewing Body, Soul, and Mind

ISBN: (paperback) 978-1-63353-623-4 , (ebook) 978-1-63353-624-1

BISAC - HEA024000 HEALTH & FITNESS / Women's Health

Printed in the United States of America

Endorsements

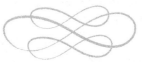

"For readers seeking to retool their life, KJ Landis offers soulful direction and encouragement. Whether you are under normal stress or suffering from tragedy, there is healing within yourself. As a hospice and bereavement professional, I see tremendous value in utilizing these stories and techniques for personal thriving after loss."
—Tracie Pyers, MSW, Medical Social Worker, Mission Hospice and Home Care

"KJ Landis' new book is compelling, with varied exercises in each chapter to help the reader work through their problems and reach positive solutions to life's challenges (workplace issues, sexual trauma, loss of loved ones, etc.). I found many of the exercises thought-provoking and so varied in style that anyone should be able to find at least one to match his or her comfort level.

She concludes her book by saying it is a testimony to Positive Psychology, and challenges us to use the information she provides to help us get unstuck, and then a natural flow will be available when new challenges arise. Indeed, this book serves as a bridge between real people with real problems, and real hope."
—Pat Madden, MPH, Social Scientist Research Coordinator, Stanford University School of Medicine

"Having as many tools as possible in our toolbox is essential for good mental health. KJ's book is one of those tools. She provides healthy mental exercises anyone can utilize when dealing with stressful issues and challenges that life can throw at us."
—Kendra Coyle, LSW, Former Social Worker at Western Psychiatric Institute & Clinic, Pittsburgh, PA

"KJ Landis' newest book Happy Healthy You is a true gift. In a world which constantly focuses us on the lack, the scarcity, and the negative, she offers a physical, mental, and spiritual guide to living a healthy life from the inside out. This is a must read for anyone who is seeking a path to spiritual renewal, healthy living, and a better life. Truly, an inspirational must read!"
—Sydney Mintz, Rabbi, Congregation Emanu-El, San Francisco

"If you ever wanted a wise coach to whisper in your ear, and cheer you up when things went wrong, here's the book for you. Happy, Healthy You engages the reader with a personal touch, well researched strategies, and stories that inspire—a true companion book on the road of your life—that you'll return to again and again."
—Kate Farrell, Librarian, Author of Word Weaving: A Teaching Sourcebook, Storyteller, Educator, Librarian, Former President, Women's National Book Association, San Francisco Chapter

"Inspirational, entertaining, and heartfelt are three great ways to describe KJ Landis' latest book. In the beginning, KJ states, I do not have a perfect life, but I do have a beautiful life. You do too. This really gets the reader thinking about the positive aspects we all can choose to focus on. With each chapter, you feel as if KJ is cheering

you on to greater things. *She is motivating you to become your superior self through realistic situations and real world exercises that can be implemented at your leisure. KJ truly does want each of us to reach for our superior selves, and it is evident through her inspirational, fun, and heartfelt tone. Do yourself a favor, reach for your yellow highlighter, read and mark up this book, dog-ear these pages, and have author and life coach KJ Landis help you along the journey of your own life. You will not regret it."*
—Suzie Roth, MLS, Research Librarian/Instructional Services Coordinator, Embry-Riddle Aeronautical University

"KJ Landis shows exhilarating enthusiasm for sharing how to drop destructive choices and habits, and then fully prepares the reader with healthier replacements. Her stories, exercises, and suggestions combine good sense, warmth, wisdom, and up-to-date approaches to optimum living."
—Melissa Riley, MLS, Self-Healing Program Coordinator, Reference Librarian, Public Library

"We are as happy as we make up our minds to be."
—Abraham Lincoln

"You may not control all the events that happen to you, but you can decide not to be reduced by them."
—Maya Angelou

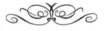

Dedicated to the elders in my tribe:

Hilda & Myron
Leota & Gary
Joseph & Mavis
and of course,
I would be nothing without my loves:
Torino, Golden, & Sage

Contents

Foreword

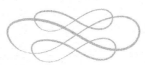

My chance meeting with KJ Landis was unrelated to her passion for health and well-being. Yet, without her saying a word about the subject, I immediately sensed a special aura and exuberance around her. I later realized I had simply picked up on her energy, which conveys the very principles for which she advocates.

On the surface one might surmise that KJ and I could not be farther apart on the healthcare spectrum. She espouses a natural approach to prevent imbalances and resolve ailments, both physical and mental. My career has been spent in the prescription pharmaceutical industry. Shouldn't we be diametrically opposed in support of our own interests and views towards quality of life and longevity? Nothing could be more incorrect, and the answer lies in the fact that I am truly thrilled KJ asked me to write the foreword for her new book.

The prescription drug industry accounts for just 10% of our country's more than one trillion dollar annual healthcare bill, while also preventing much more expensive hospitalizations every day. I sincerely believe it is also a fact that following KJ's teachings can dramatically reduce the incidence of hospitalization as well as the excessive use of prescription drugs. This is good news for everyone, and good for our economy in terms of individual productivity and taxpayer burden.

KJ's expertise extends to two primary areas – in her first book, the foods and beverages we choose to consume, and in this, her newest publication, the mental perspective. Our minds play a critical role in every aspect of our overall health. Oncologists I've met acknowledge that 50% or more of the success for any treatment outcome has to do with the cancer patient having a positive mental attitude. I am convinced that a majority of the prescription drugs used for conditions such as anxiety/depression, as well as obesity and diabetes, could be minimized or eliminated by following KJ's simple and realistic lifestyle recommendations.

Of all the guidance KJ offers in her new book, the part which resonates with me most is both powerful and succinct. "Suspend your own negative belief system," she writes. Most of us might not even recognize we operate within a paradigm of negativity, but correcting that can open up an entirely new way of not just living, but enjoying life. KJ's books detail pathways to helping create a happier, fitter nation, while eliminating the need to always rely on prescription medicines as a first resort.

And finally, as she writes, "Be grateful." Be grateful for everything and to everyone, as we are diminished when we take even a moment of life for granted.

—Robert G. Partridge, Head of Marketing and Public Relations, Cutanea Life Sciences, A New Prescription Dermatology Company

Preface

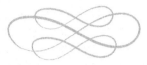

I do not have a perfect life, but I do have a beautiful life. You do too. We do not realize this all of the time, especially when we are in the whirlwind of our daily duties.

My first book, *Superior Self* dealt with mind, body, and spiritual paths to physical health and wellness, what foods and movements assist us in vitality as we age, and preventive healing therapies through foods. It also showed us where to turn to for motivation and inspiration.

After *Superior Self* was published, I received many emails and letters inquiring about how to gain more willpower to achieve life goals, especially after going through a myriad of personal traumas including depression, stress, money woes, childhood abuse and all the issues we can encounter in our life's path.

The protocols, dos, and don'ts were relatively simple, but the mental fortitude was a struggle for most folks. The psychological barriers were just too much to bear. Once again, people turned to me for help.

This book aims to give you all the tools to create a happy healthy life, full of vibrancy and vitality. I want you to experience physical health that is optimal, rather than normal or average. I want you to let go of past struggles that may have kept you weeping at night, not sleeping, sleeping too much, not eating, binge eating, or perhaps turning to alcohol, drugs, or unsafe sex.

Whatever we humans go through during this precious time on earth, there are answers and tools. My toolkit is waiting for you to open it. Keep reading my friends. It is my hopeful effort to create here a life map that you can travel through to help heal the wounds caused by the things that get us stuck in the first place. There are examples here of human trauma and drama. There are examples here of how we can see the heavy challenges and every day constant pressures in new ways. We can see them as springboards to heal, thrive, and become our most authentic selves, our superior selves. We will learn how these folks reacted to their lifestyle situations, how they finally shifted to a different method of recovery and rebounding, and from that learning, we will figure out a way to maneuver our *own* struggles and our *own* outcomes in positive ways.

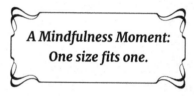

A Mindfulness Moment:
One size fits one.

This is not a one size fits all kind of book. This is a one size fits one kind of book. Everybody receives information in different ways. I'm fully aware that some of my readers will skip through the chapters to see which stories and exercises resonate with them. Feel free to meander through this work.

Having options is nice. Having an option that fits in with your ideals is even better. Having too many options is sometimes detrimental and causes us to procrastinate. Think about the options we have every day that prevent us from healing from our deep rooted problems. "I'll get to it after shopping, errands, cleaning, my TV show, cooking, eating, etc." The business of being busy can be a way of running away.

We all are guilty of this procrastination tactic. A good starting point is recognizing that *busy-ness* and consumption do not feed our true motivation, and they do not assist us in reaching our end goals. Then we can choose a plan (the exercises in this book), face one fear or problem, and settle that ONE. Choose no more than three ways to attack it, but at first, do *one* exercise only. I always encourage folks to keep a little notebook to work in. Take it everywhere with you. Then, when the *aha* moment arrives, you can acknowledge it and document it. Well done. The notebook will be your success book (your *YES* book.).

During my years as a friend, confidante, and professional coach, I have helped people during their journeys to wellness. It has always required taking a holistic and multifaceted approach. Their stories give examples of a variety of problems and a variety of solutions. Individuals, being as unique as they are, will have different journeys to recovering from personal tragedies. It's all good. And, no, you do not have to be a complete @#$%up to receive benefit from this book.

Please note that I am not a medical professional, nor do I play one on television. I am not an expert in the field of psychology. I do not, in any way, consider that a limitation to my credentials. My qualifications are not bound by the often slow-moving pace of information and trickle-down effect in much of academia, nor are they limited by membership in professional organizations or lack thereof.

The content in this book is for informational use only. It is not intended for diagnosis or treatment of any medical condition. Please seek out your own health practitioner before embarking upon any new lifestyle change. I have, however, done years of research, coaching, soul searching, and self experimentation in order to bring you the most relevant and accurate information. As the science changes, so must we.

We will see how folks process through their troubles, as well as provide other options to consider when healing from serious life events. The stories here are autobiographical fiction, a combination of my own life experiences on earth for more than fifty years, adding in my great imagination, coaching experiences, and research. Except for my name, all of the names have been changed. The purpose of writing these stories is to be clear with the reader on how to get un-stuck, how to move forward in life goals, and how to shed pain once and for all. If you reach in and use the multiple modalities provided here for you in this loving toolkit, you will find a *Happy, Healthy You.*

Fix me now! Instant gratification

We live in a society now that has a sense of immediacy. We expect instant solutions and gratifications. The truth is, we cannot expect 80% benefits from 20% efforts. We must do 100% of the work in order to receive 100% of the benefits in life.

We cannot put our own expiration date on how long it takes to reach our goals. We cannot say that we are going to give it only a few weeks and then if it doesn't work we will quit, and continue to live *less than*. Most people quit working on themselves because it doesn't work fast enough. In our modern society we have developed a sense of entitlement that says we deserve to feel better in a short period of time because we *want to* and because we put in the effort consistently (for those few weeks). We must change this mentality. We must continue to make efforts in healing from our rut, however long that may be. When we figure out the root of our rut, we may take steps forward in healing and growing. Don't give up on yourselves. There are so many people around you who are there to support you. There are professionals in the healing arts that are available as well. It does take time. You are worth the time and the effort.

I'm not saying we should not take efficient measures and shortcuts in mundane, everyday tasks, but in the core values, deep goals, and intense passions of our lives, we must make a full effort in order to reach full satisfaction. If we take shortcuts on the little things, we then have more energy and time to devote to the things that mean the most to us. Some things in life you can't rush, you can't cram for, and you can't fake.

When was the last time you felt completely confident in your own shoes? When were you wholly grounded, certain of who you were, knew instinctively what great things you had to offer the world, and knew your faults too? When was this all clear in your head and heart? Take some moments now to ponder your answers to these questions.

When my son was in second grade, I volunteered to create a project for the school auction. I am a photographer who adores shooting real film portraits in black and white. So, I created an **I AM** project with the children. They wrote on a big piece of paper in big letters: **I AM**... Then they finished the sentence with a statement about who they were at their core; their beliefs, their feelings, and their attributes. Some students had to think long and hard before coming up with something that rang true to their hearts. I noticed that *not one* child wrote something negative or self deprecating on their papers. On his paper, my son wrote, "I AM a happy spirit."

That photo still sits prominently on his shelves.

An Invitation: I am

A Mindfulness Moment: I am the most important person in my life.

Breathe deeply. Go back to a powerful, confident time of your life in your mind. What was it that made you so sure of yourself? Write down I AM... Write those things down. Take a selfie with the list. Print it. Put it somewhere where you can glance at it daily. Start your journey to awesomeness there. You rock! Even if it was a long time ago, like when you were a toddler, you had a unique flow that said to the world, "Here I am. You can't hold *me* back."

This is where I want us to travel throughout this book. We will learn how to dissect trauma and drama. We will use what we learn for life's enhancement at best, and at the very least, we will understand ourselves better. The many struggles humans suffer from can be a springboard to greatness. In the coming chapters, I have created written exercises and role play activities, similar to the one you just completed. They will allow you to hone your skills in being completely honest with yourself. Real change can occur if we trust the process.

We do not have to permit our past to control our future. It is information, that's all. We do not have to allow the past to continue to stop...everything. You are here, now. You picked up this book at the right time and for the right reasons. I believe nothing is by accident. In this book, you will realize that we cannot give up our past completely, because it is those experiences that built up our personality, strengths, and character as well.

We must, however, get to the present, and that's where we want to be. Let's break through the barriers together. After all, everywhere you go, there you are.

At the end of the book, let us meet a *Happy, Healthy You.*

Acknowledgements

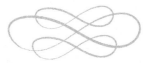

My heartfelt gratitude pours out to the San Francisco Public Library. The library has provided me with the many materials used in my work over the years, as well as giving me a welcome platform for my wellness workshops. I have been a fan for years and will continue to support them, as they have done me a great service.

Thank you to Mango Publishing for taking a chance on me and my passions. I spent the first half of my life absorbing life lessons. I dedicate the second half of my life to giving through the world of words. With Brenda Knight as my editor, ally, angel, and mentor, I have grown in leaps and bounds. Thank you, Brenda. I am grateful to the CEO, Chris, and to the marketing and design team for working so patiently with me, as I didn't know anything about that side of the business or the tech stuff. Heck, my kids had to teach me how to type and create a website a couple of years ago. I thought FB meant fall back.

Thank you to my tribe of email and personal clients on the World Wide Web, as well as those of you who are in my face. Thank you to my followers on all of my social media and to the readers out there who take the time to give me feedback and ask real, pertinent questions that will help transform your lives for the better when you do apply the principles from my books to your own worlds. You all have put your trust and hope into my hands, and I do not take that lightly.

And finally, thank you to my family and friends. You have been my sounding board in the wee hours of the morning and my rocks of strength when my own personal $#!+ hit the fan. I pray I have not turned you all off from the prospect of writing your own book one day. It really is a remarkable process that is reminiscent of the yellow brick road. I love you all.

Introduction

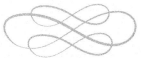

My Wish and Prayer That You Get Unstuck

Are you living with chronic pain? Do you worry that nobody really understands your physical or emotional suffering? Are you so busy taking care of other people and *things* that you have brushed your own dreams aside? Have people told you that your dreams are just plain crazy at your age? Are you feeling a little overwhelmed all the time or close to the edge? Do you feel stuck? Have you been hurt so many times, that hurt is all you know, and it is your expectation of others' impact on you?

You are not alone. Every horrific story you can tell me that's happened to you has happened to someone else in this world. Just like we all have doppelgangers somewhere who look exactly like us, someone has felt what you have felt and has experienced close to what you have experienced, some time in this lifetime. Think about it. There are an awful lot of people on planet Earth. I am not minimizing your pain, suffering, or experiences, but I am telling you that you can decide to not let it hold you back anymore.

You have the God-given ability to turn things around, and to take action in order to become your superior self. You will do more than bounce back to your normal self. You will become the extraordinary person who has been glowing softly inside of you the whole time you thought you couldn't, shouldn't, or wouldn't...

It is my wish and prayer that you do not remain stuck in a beautifully, ornate bird cage, singing your glorious, heavenly song, looking and sounding so moving that it brings tears to the eyes of anyone passing by, yet *still* inside that bird cage.

When we hold on to bitterness, anger, and hatred, it serves no one, especially not ourselves. Somehow we need to figure out how to turn it around so we do not keep living on auto pilot, and remain paralyzed in our current situation. OK, so you were screwed over in your life. People took advantage of you. You made poor choices and suffered the consequences. *What now?*

"Self pity in its early stages is as snug as a feather mattress. Only when it hardens does it become uncomfortable."
—Maya Angelou, author

Here is an opportunity to go deeper into what happened to you, and to organically produce a different outcome. As with all of life's *aha* moments, these lessons will take effort on your part. The true understanding may not come immediately after completing the soul work. As someone very close to me once said, "You cannot speed up understanding."[1]

I am often referred to as a friend, an ally, a mother-type, and a nurturer. People trust me with their most intimate, secret, vulnerable, scary, and never before shared stories and thoughts. My friends and clients know I have created a safe space for them to purge their troubles from their body and soul. Together we pick up the pieces, communicate honestly, create true connection, and create an invitation to change. We rebuild a shiny, strong *Happy, Healthy You*, one baby step at a time, but it does take time. I'm immensely grateful for that trust. When I use my role play or writing exercises to assist in healing, I always feel a lesson is there for me as well.

I'm not a medical professional of any type. I am a good listener and a creative type of person. Perhaps my nurturing character and studies in childhood development have made me the type of support person that I am.

In the self-reflective exercises you will find throughout this book, there are no right or wrong answers. They are for your heart, mind, notebook and eyes only, so feel completely at ease being open and honest with yourself.

Have you ever wanted to physically destroy your negative thoughts? The *Negative Thought Pot* is a tool I use for my family and for my wellness workshops. We write our written fears and negative self-judgments on strips of paper, roll them up tightly into little scrolls, and place them in a clay pot. We then set the paper on fire, literally destroying those thoughts. Those thoughts and worries have no more power over us. To me, fear equals hate. Whether it is a tiny fear or a grand one, it is still a form of self hate. I say, burn it up.

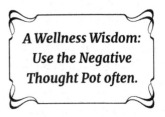

A Wellness Wisdom: Use the Negative Thought Pot often.

During the written exercises in this book, if you feel someone may intrude on your personal growth and privacy by looking though your journals or tiny notebook in any way, feel free to set fire to the written work in the notebook page by page. Tear out the pages and destroy them in the *Negative Thought Pot*. Do this only after meditating upon and learning from your answers.

Inside this book you will learn the origin of how and why some of us pick up bad habits or cling to less than ideal routines after crises in our lives. You will learn how the role of nutrition affects every aspect of our mental and physical health. You will learn about the endocrine system, the home of hormones, and then how hormones affect every system in the body. You will be exposed to the power of self-care through restorative practices. You will learn how to use daily affirmations for positive outcomes. You will learn how to use silence as a healer through different modalities. You will see how epigenetics relate to genetics and figure out how we can alter our gene expression to become the best version of ourselves, our happy, healthy selves.

Some of the themes I just mentioned are also discussed in my first book.[2] Here, we will dig way deeper into utilizing those techniques, and discover other tools for letting go and for moving forward. We will find new answers to old questions.

It is my personal belief that we chose to come down here to earth from some other side (heaven, spirit world, or dimension), and that when we were on the other side, we chose to have these challenges here on earth. I think we made a sort of agreement with the universe (God, angels, All That Is). This is my belief only. I do not believe that we choose to be obese, chronically ill, afflicted with cancer, raped, abused, neglected, put down, criticized, etc., but we did choose to have some things to work on so that we could grow deeply in our soul-spot. Maybe it was a subconscious or a super-conscious decision.

I want you to face your superior self sooner rather than later. I don't want you to *get it* at the moment of your death. I want you to get it now (or at least by the end of this book).

Feeling good is worth it. Feeling great is worth the challenge, the process, the journey, and the efforts.

I invite you to lose the baggage and blame. Face your superior self. Embrace a *Happy, Healthy You.*

Chapter One

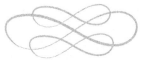

The Root of the Rut ~ The Inside Out Approach to Healing

What is a life rut? A life rut is like supergluing your feet to the hardwood floor in the gym after your high school basketball game. Everyone else goes home, but you are stuck there all night. You are tired and you are hungry. You want to pee, lie down, and do something different, but you can't. You don't know how. This is all you know until you figure out how to get help and where this gluey mess all started. How do we get stuck in a life rut in the first place? It begins with the subtle or not so subtle experience of feeling *less than*. Perhaps, when you were really young, like toddler age to seven or so, you were made to feel that you were not good enough at something. It may not have always been expressed blatantly, but you may have perceived this message anyway.

How do we recognize those times in our lives when we are in a rut?

One symptom of a life rut may be that we stay at the same position at work for years, do the work of our supervisors, and do not ask for recognition, a raise, or a new position for far too long. What are we really afraid of? Where does this come from? Another symptom of a rut may be when we make the decision (over and over) to choose vegetables over fried foods when eating away from home, but then within a couple of weeks find ourselves back at the happy hour buffet eating the fried mozzarella with coworkers because we allow ourselves to sabotage our promises to ourselves. Whose path are we on anyway? We are practicing the same negative behaviors over and over again and we are not serving our higher purpose in life, or our immediate promises to ourselves. That is a rut. What and where does the rut come from originally?

June's Story: feeling unrooted was the root of her rut

My friend June could not keep a job as a butcher. She was a fabulous master carver, and all the chefs in her city loved her sing-song voice and her masterful skills with the knife. They followed her around from butcher shop to butcher shop, because she only worked for the finest places, and the meat she carved was of the highest quality. Truth be told, June bucked authority like no one I had ever seen. She either quit or was fired from 16 butcher shops within six years. Over steaming cups of coffee, I had a heart to heart with June one day, asking her why she could not keep a job she obviously loved so much.

"The root of my rut is I have no roots. I mean, I *feel* like I have no roots. I was adopted as an infant from an orphanage in Thailand and my parents here kept telling me how lucky I was to have them, how grateful I should be. I am grateful, and I love them, but I feel like something is missing. I don't feel grounded. I know I am in a rut. I keep doing the same thing over and over again. I recognize I am self-sabotaging my career, which I love. I want to find out who my birth parents are. I want to feel my roots or have closure and tie up the roots once and for all. I want to meet my birth parents if they are alive and have a connection. I want to see the orphanage in Thailand, if it still exists."

June saved her money from the time we spoke and within six months she had enough for a one month trip to Thailand to fulfill her dreams. She came back to the United States an empowered woman, after having seen her birthplace and met her birth parents for the first time. They were dirt poor, they had three other children to care for, and had no way of caring for her. They could not afford birth control either, but clearly loved each other. June was born in June, hence the name. She met her siblings for the first time. Two other siblings were born after June, and they too were brought to the orphanage and put up for adoption. She emails her family members regularly now, and has kept the same butcher position with the same company for three years. She feels grounded and whole at last. Even though she is in one place, she is definitely unstuck and out of her rut of either quitting or being fired from jobs. She is at peace with herself because she knows where she comes from.

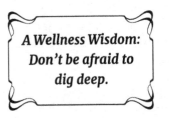

> *A Wellness Wisdom:*
> *Don't be afraid to*
> *dig deep.*

Did your parents or teachers imply that straight A's were the only grades worth striving for? Mine did. Were you pushed to be the star athlete, a musical prodigy, or an ace at something? Were you constantly being compared to others in your family who were around the same age? If you didn't live up to those expectations, perhaps you put yourself down internally, even if your elders didn't criticize you openly. If you don't unlock the cause of the emotional distress, you will likely end up chasing your own tail for years. Elements of feeling judged by others *or* negatively judging ourselves can have a profound effect on our mental and physical health.

My Story: food equaled love - and I was loved a lot (the root of my rut)

When my grades were all A's, my parents showered me with food, love, and praise, and shared my accolades with our relatives and their adult friends. The longer I maintained my A average (my entire K-12 education), the more they treated me to meals out, desserts, candies, and treats. Boy did that backfire. At age 12, I stood five feet two inches tall and weighed 173 pounds. **Food equaled love**. So, when I finally got it together on the food front, emotionally, my mom and dad viewed my clean eating as a rejection of their love, even though analytically they realized it was a smart thing their obese daughter was doing (by changing her eating habits).

I did not want to hurt their feelings and reject their years of love and accolades as I was learning how to eat real food without processed carbohydrates, refined sugars, hydrolyzed oils, chemical additives, and preservatives.

Food equaled love. Let's go deeper into the root of my rut. Specifically, the kinds of foods that were just coming out in the late 1960s and 1970s were packaged convenience foods, made to last on the store shelves longer, made to be cooked in the oven or microwave within minutes, and made to help make a busy, working mom and wife's life easier. My mother was very busy, as I was the youngest of five children.

My parents grew up during the Depression era and they had to deal with less food and more day to day survival issues than I did while growing up. In their eyes, when I rejected their abundance of convenient and modern foods, I was saying *no* to their success and their struggles of that era. Basically, I was rejecting their memories without knowing it. It felt to them like I was silently belittling their ordeal during those times.

Our Relationship With Our Body: start here

A common rut in the United States of America is our uneven relationship with our bodies. Our skewed thinking between mind and body becomes our behavior around food. I was not alone in my behavior during the era of the snack food, fast food, convenient food, and junk food boom of the 1970s and 1980s. The root of this behavioral rut may start with our relationship with our body. We may be uncomfortable with the body changes that occurred when we were in our preteens. The hormonal changes made our scent, body shape, hair, and emotions change. We were not in control of our food choices while we were kids. Our parents made all the food choices for us, for our own good (or so they thought). If they were listening to the mainstream dietary advice of the time, they were following the Standard American Diet. The packaged, processed foods included in that recommended eating style contributed to our hormonal, metabolic, and behavioral downfall. Those foods are specifically produced so as to make us want more of them.

When I was fifty pounds heavier, I was so happy to find unusual earrings, or to find shoes that were on sale that fit my size 11 feet. I usually focused on my face or feet in full length mirrors. It was way too painful to look at my entire body in a mirror, head to toe. Coincidentally, my customers at the restaurant always commented on my earrings or shoes too.

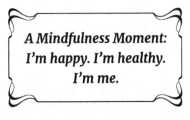

A Mindfulness Moment:
I'm happy. I'm healthy.
I'm me.

After digging deeply into my past, I wrote down my less than perfect thoughts about myself that said I wasn't good enough. I wished I was one of those people who didn't think about food. I wished I was one of those people who forgets to eat. (My first boyfriend was one of those types.) I wished I was one of those people who just goes without food without realizing it. I burned those wishes and thoughts up in the *Negative Thought Pot* with great satisfaction. Then I was able to move on. I was finally successful in my wellness goals. Months later, I was able to enjoy my full reflection with self-love. Other people reacted to my shift in positive ways too. What I thought about, I brought about.

For me, my downfall *and* my healing arrived with food. Food was my personal starting point. Why? If I feed every cell in my body with the most nourishing, healing, life-giving, vital foods, the cell centers are fed. That, in turn, feeds my brain and body, and I have energy, creativity, and a positive attitude. I truly feel vibrant and vital, with flexibility, agility, and strength. I make choices that are smarter too. I am reading and remembering facts from my research better. My blood work is now in the optimal range rather than in the normal range. I am a happy, healthy me.

This is an example of one root problem that is causing various ruts in the United States of America and beyond. We are the most obese nation on earth, with chronic diseases and conditions related to obesity, that include anxiety, addictions, depression, and other psychological illnesses. Ironically, we have the most diet protocols and supplements for the problem of obesity. Yet, we remain stuck on the hamster wheel. "If only I lost *X* number of pounds of fat, my life would be perfect. I would be happy and healthy. Mr. or Ms. Right would fall in love with me and we would live happily ever after."

Please allow me to pop the sugary, sweet, and fake bubble you have been sold by the diet industry. Real food works. When you get off the pills and potions you will have to learn how to transition into a real food eating lifestyle for the long term anyway, so I encourage folks to start their journey to body, soul, and mind wellness by eating real food.

I have devoted years researching up to date studies on fat loss, hormones, and how nutrient dense foods relate to mental wellness and emotions. My recent area of interest is in studying the function of the intestines, the prebiotics that feed the probiotics which live there, and how the rest of our body and attitude is influenced by a happy or unhappy gut. I have learned about the importance of human touch, essential oil therapy, movement, restorative practices, humor, playing, and connecting daily with people we love. I am passionate about teaching others how to build a tribe of support when changing their lifestyle for the better. I encourage others to seek out and build a community of like minded individuals.

During my years as a life and wellness coach I have developed a shift in eating that slowly takes us away from the Standard American Diet and leads us to the most nutrient-dense eating style that I know. This is the real food eating style I mentioned above. I advocate eating food in the form closest to how God made it, without added colorings, preservatives, or chemicals. Foods like cheese puffs, with their hot pink or orange hue, are not found in nature, either in color, flavor, or texture.

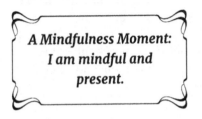

A Mindfulness Moment: I am mindful and present.

This shift is not a diet. There are no points and no calories to count. There are no comparisons of carbs to fats to proteins. As stated earlier, this is a nourishing real foods eating lifestyle for the long term meant to sustain and enhance your total wellness in mind, body, and soul.

This guide will help with cravings for junk food and sugary treats. It may not be easy at first, because it may be different than what you have been eating to live thus far. With time, trust in the process, and patience you will find yourself not wanting the foods of the past. They no longer serve you. There is no time limit as to how long each step may take to master. It will take precision. Each day, be mindful and present with each meal. Be precise. That means focus on just that one day, that one meal, that one moment. Say in your head, over and over again, "Just for today." It will help keep you from feeling overwhelmed. It is entirely up to you. As with any lifestyle change, please check with your health care practitioner before embarking upon *Superior Self's Guide to Wellness from Within.*

In my first book, *Superior Self,* I shared a shift in eating called **Superior Self's Guide to Wellness from Within**. I believe, without a doubt, that if we take care of ourselves with basic, good, real foods, our brains, hearts, and bodies will function in the best way possible for us. This allows us to receive dynamic health and a dynamic life. We will think more clearly. We will sleep better. Our hormonal system will be in better balance. We will heal from drama and trauma with fewer struggles. The intestines, or gut, are now being called the second brain. We need to feed it well. With real food, we may have more of those *aha* moments. We will be able to reach for our superior selves. We will be happy and healthy.

Superior Self's Guide to Wellness from Within is a system of small shifts toward eating the most nutrient dense foods possible. These shifts can be made weekly, monthly, or you can take as long as you need to take, as long as they are made with 100% commitment. The steps in the guide must be done sequentially, and they must build upon each other in order to be successful. Eat local, organic, and in-season foods when you can find them and when it fits your budget to buy them. Here we go!

Superior Self's Guide to Wellness from Within[3]

The plan can be used week by week (or month by month, or longer).

I suggest:

Step 1- Increase water to a gallon a day. Remember to go slowly.

Here's why: Water consumption lubricates our entire body from the inside. It makes the joints less achy and the skin supple and fresh looking. Water assists the digestive system, moving food and their nutrients through the body. Increased water consumption aids in relieving constipation. Fat cells increase or decrease in size, but most humans still have the same number of fat cells in their bodies that they have had since toddlerhood (unless we surgically remove them). When changing food intake to healthier choices, fat cells may very well shrink. Water consumption helps us sweat and urinate more. The more water that goes in, the more water goes out. Drinking lots of water also rids the body of toxins.

When we drink lots of water, we may find ourselves satisfied with less food and our impulses to eat junk food fade away. With more water consumption, we can identify if we are truly hungry, or emotionally and socially hungry. I add yummy fresh flavors to pitchers of water in order to help get a gallon of water into my body. I put sliced strawberries and mint leaves in one pitcher, sliced tomatoes and basil leaves in one pitcher, sliced cucumbers and cantaloupe in one pitcher, and lemon, lime, and orange slices in another pitcher. I was at Whole Foods recently and saw a sixteen ounce bottle of cinnamon stick/apple slice water for $6.99. I add electrolyte powder or a pinch of Pink Himalayan salt to the water jug to add extra minerals to my day. Sometimes I have to negotiate with my children about who gets the last glass of water because the water jugs are so delicious.

Step 2- Give up all wheat and gluten containing products and continue to drink a gallon of water a day.

Here's why: Wheat and gluten containing products are high on the list of foods that are common allergens to which people are highly sensitive. Most folks do not even know they are sensitive to these foods until they eliminate them from their lifestyle and see remarkable improvements. Wheat and gluten containing products are in many highly processed foods. Most commercial salad dressings have wheat and gluten in them, as well as a host of scientific sounding flavors and additives. Wheat and gluten act like glue in the body and make food "stick to our ribs." Wheat is one of the crops that has been most altered by the farming industries.

Wheat can be inflammatory in the body's systems. Consistent, chronic inflammation from highly processed, gluten-filled convenience foods can cause obesity and conditions related to obesity. Most people are sensitive to wheat, but don't realize it. Yet, when they follow my guide and give it up, they find aches, pains, gas, acne, eczema, and bloating fading away. Here are the most common foods containing wheat and gluten:

- All Wheat Types
- Bread
- Cereals
- Pasta
- Cookies
- Pastries
- Pies
- Commercial Salad Dressings
- Commercial Sauces
- Pre-packaged Meals
- Frozen Complete Meals
- Soy Products
- Couscous
- Crackers
- Beer
- Some Oats

- Rye
- Barley
- Gravy
- Cakes
- Muffins
- Flour Tortillas
- Modified Food Starch
- Some Lunch Meats and Some Hot Dogs
- Some Seasoned Chips
- Some Imitation Seafood and Fish
- Malt
- Matzo
- Some Candies
- Bouillon Cubes
- Some Croutons and Bread Crumbs

The takeaway message here is that knowledge is power. Start to read ingredient labels if you buy things in boxes. Better yet, have fun in the kitchen and begin to make your own gluten free and wheat free versions of old favorites.

If you miss wheat and gluten containing processed foods, there are alternatives. If you love pizza, try a gluten free flour to make your crust. Most restaurants offer a gluten free version nowadays. For salad dressings, I suggest making your own. They are easier than you think. Here is a recipe to get you started on the wheat free and gluten free path. Not only is this recipe wheat free and gluten free, it is completely grain free.

CAULIFLOWER CRUST PIZZA

INGREDIENTS:

- 2 bags frozen riced cauliflower or 1 giant head of cauliflower
- 3 eggs
- 1/2 cup coconut flour (or optionally almond, tapioca, or chestnut flour)
- 1/2 cup heavy whipping cream or coconut milk
- 2 Tablespoons extra virgin olive oil
- 1/2 cup butter or coconut oil
- 1 cup shredded mozzarella cheese
- 1 cup hard Parmesan cheese, grated by hand
- 1/2 cup nutritional yeast flakes
- salt and pepper to taste
- garlic powder to taste
- dried oregano to taste
- 8 oz. sliced, sundried tomatoes in olive oil
- optional toppings: tomatoes, zucchini, olives, spinach, broccoli, mushrooms, leeks, and other family favorites.

DIRECTIONS:

1. Cook riced cauliflower on stovetop according to directions on the bag. If using the whole head of cauliflower, mash with potato masher.

2. Roll mashed cauliflower in paper towels until all the moisture is out of it.

3. Add eggs, garlic, oregano, and nutritional yeast flakes. Mix thoroughly.

4. Add salt, pepper, and butter or coconut oil. Mix thoroughly.

5. Add coconut flour and mix thoroughly.

6. Add half of the mozzarella and half of the Parmesan.

7. Mix with hands.

8. On a large cookie sheet, spread olive oil on parchment paper.

9. Spread mixture evenly over parchment paper.

10. Bake for 30 minutes at 400° or until bottom of crust is golden brown.

11. Take out of oven and spread the sun-dried tomatoes evenly with a little of their own olive oil.

12. Add remaining cheeses and veggies of your choice.

13. Bake in the oven for another 35 minutes at 400° or until edges are crispy and dark brown.

14. Be creative! Add meats, different sauces, cheeses, and try vegetables you have never tried before.

Step 3- Give up all grains and continue to drink a gallon of water a day.

Here's why: All grains have to be processed in order to be edible. Those wheat berries, as well as corn, millet, rye, barley, or oats must be picked, dried, split open, or ground. Then we must cook them in order to digest them. The smaller and finer the grind, the higher the glycemic index. Extra fine bakers' flour has a much higher glycemic index (how much the food affects the blood sugar level) than a wheat berry in its original form even though it is the same wheat. This causes glucose and insulin levels to spike during digestion. The high energy spike is followed by a crash, and then low energy ensues. So, we may reach for another high carbohydrate snack to raise our blood sugar levels again. It is a vicious cycle. The sugar in the blood stream is processed by the liver and if we are not using up the energy right away by exercising, it is readily turned to fat, the kind of fat we do not need or want.

All plant matter turns to glucose in the bloodstream. Cereal, spinach, an orange, or pineapple juice all will be converted into sugar. The rate of absorption is fast or slow depending upon the amount of fiber in the food. Spinach has the most fiber and lowest glycemic index. If you miss starch and want an easy substitute for *starchy grains* I suggest:

- Yams

- Sweet Potatoes

- Butternut Squash

- Acorn Squash

- White Potatoes

- Quinoa

- Coconut Oil Prepared Potato Chips

- Olive Oil Prepared Potato Chips

- Coconut Oil Prepared Sweet Potato Chips

- Olive Oil Prepared Sweet Potato Chips

- Kale Chips
- Plantain Chips
- Kabocha Squash
- Heirloom Carrots
- Parsnips

- Chestnuts
- Turnips
- Rutabaga
- French Fries, Cooked in Healthy Oil
- Sweet Potato Fries, Cooked in Healthy Oil

For baking I suggest using tapioca, chestnut, coconut, or almond flour.

Step 4- Reduce fruits to one to two times a day, while continuing with previous dietary shifts (i.e., no grains and a gallon of water each day).

Here's why: Fruits these days are sweeter than the ancient wild ones grown without agricultural practices. Thousands of years ago, fruit was eaten when in season and ripe. Our ancestors did not get to eat fruit very often. Today's fruit growers have perfected uniform colors and sizes in fruit crops. They are also grown to be sweet on purpose. This causes insulin spikes and cravings for more sweet tasting things.

The whole point of **Step 4 is to *get real*.** Most of us do have a sugar problem, but do not see it as such. If you say that you hardly ever eat ice cream or dessert, I believe you. Then we may go over your daily eating diary. I look at breakfast and see coffee with half and half and a plain bagel with butter, a nonfat bagel at that. The bagel turns into glucose in the blood stream because it is highly processed white flour. Then at 10a.m. you had some nonfat strawberry yogurt and carrot sticks and cheese. The strawberry yogurt has added sugar and extra milk sugar to make the nonfat parts taste like milk again.

Lunch was a tuna salad sandwich with veggies on whole wheat bread with light mayonnaise and chopped veggies on the side. Mayonnaise is usually made from canola oil which is heated to toxic temperatures to release the oil from the rapeseed. There is a lot of sugar added to mayonnaise. The bread is highly processed and full of gluten and will turn to glucose in the blood stream. You sipped on diet lemonade to top off the meal and added a non fat frozen yogurt for dessert. Sugar substitutes, which are chemically derived, make the brain think we had sugar and cause the liver to react as if we have eaten sugar, so then we crave more sugar.

Dinner was at a chain restaurant where they serve menus with calories next to each item. You had the "lite"-fare. What they forgot to share was some key information about the ingredients, like the toxic canola oil, gluten, wheat, and soy, and the 16 teaspoons of sugar in the commercial salad dressing they used on your "lite" salad. The menu omitted the amount of high fructose corn syrup in the BBQ sauce on your breast of pumped up, hormonally dosed chicken. The food industry fooled you (and me) for years, but now we are educating ourselves so we may live optimally and pain free from the inside out, so that we may renew ourselves, body, soul, and mind.

This is the *get real* moment when I tell you again, "I think we need to reduce your fruits and eventually we will reduce your sugar. Your cravings for carbohydrates from processed foods and sugary foods will fade with time. You have to trust the process and honor your precise efforts."

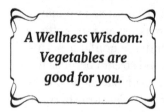

A Wellness Wisdom: Vegetables are good for you.

Step 5- Reduce fruits to one to two servings a week.

Here's why: Once we are able to conquer the fruit reduction to 1-2 times a day, it is time to lessen our fruit intake even more. I suggest the following substitutes for fruit:

- Carrots
- Raw Shredded Coconut
- Fennel
- Sweet Potatoes
- Sweet Peppers

- Winter Squash
- Raw Chocolate
- Cheeses
- Nuts and their Butters

Reach for high fat foods instead of high sugar foods. This will keep blood sugar levels more even throughout the day. You may find yourself not wanting fruits or sweet vegetables very often after curtailing sweet produce consumption for a few weeks.

Step 6- Change your oils and fats to only healthy dietary fats like extra virgin olive oil, raw grass-fed dairy, grass fed fatty meats, avocados, raw tree nuts and butters, and minimally processed coconut products.

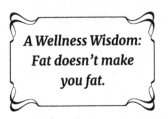

A Wellness Wisdom: Fat doesn't make you fat.

Here's why: Fats and oils from minimally processed foods will provide energy for hours, and they produce a super satisfying, creamy mouth feel. My favorite afternoon pick-me-up is raw butter, raw milk cheese, and homemade sugar free preserves on a grain-free flax cracker. The high omega-3 oils and lots of healthy fats provide mental focus and clarity.

I eat a high fat diet and stay slim. Healthy fats help us absorb the vitamins, minerals, and phytochemicals from the vegetables we eat with them. I put raw butter or extra virgin olive oil on my steamed and oven roasted veggies, my grass fed and grass finished meats, my wild fish, and my wild caught seafood. The only nut I eat roasted is the peanut because it is actually a bean (most beans and legumes are better absorbed by the body when cooked).

Fats are not found in nature all by themselves. They are bound to something else. For example, meat has fat in and around it; avocados have flesh with both fiber and fat, and olives do as well. Butter, cheeses and oils are made after milking, crushing, fermenting, and so forth. We don't go walking in the woods and suddenly come upon a clearing and say to our hiking partner, "Look, a field of butter! Let's pick it and eat it!" Oils and fats are best absorbed and utilized by the body when eaten in their whole form. The body is natural and whole. The whole food form is natural and whole. Natural understands natural. The whole food form is minimally processed when compared to the oil form so the nutrients are more bioavailable to the body. When available and affordable, I encourage folks to eat avocado as well as consume avocado oil. I suggest you eat olives and enjoy extra virgin olive oil. Does this make sense?

Here are a few oils and fats I recommend:

Extra Virgin Olive Oil: Use at room temperature and toss in after the veggies are done or use when roasting foods in the oven. If sautéing on the stovetop keep food temperatures less than 450 degrees so that the heat does not cause smoking and the molecules of the fat do not change. When oils and fat molecules get overheated, past their smoke point, the good qualities of the dietary fat are lost and the healthy fat becomes something else entirely.

Grape Seed Oil: Use as a neutral oil for any recipe because it has no flavor or odor. It is great for salad dressings and sauces. It is mostly poly-unsaturated fat and should not be heated, even though it has a high smoke point.

Coconut Oil and Palm Oil: Use at any temperature, but be aware that it will harden at room temperature. I use coconut oil for my skin and hair, as well as for cooking at high heat, making baked goods, frying, thickening sauces, oiling the furniture, whitening my teeth, and more.

Butter, rendered lard, duck fat, rendered beef tallow, and rendered chicken fat: Use freely at varied temperatures, sticking to grass fed and raw, unpasteurized butter when you can afford it and when you can find it in your area. These all have a high temperature smoke point.

Ghee: Use ghee if you are sensitive to the milk proteins in butter. It has the good fats with most of the casein milk protein skimmed off of the top.

Nut and Seed Oils: Depending on the nut or seed, the smoke point and the mono-unsaturated, poly-unsaturated, or saturated bond of the fat molecule is different for each. Please do your research before cooking. When in doubt, toss oils on after cooking for flavor and health benefits.

If you want to dig deeper into the world of dietary fats, I highly recommend looking at:

http://www.healthyeatsreal.com
http://www.eatnakednow.com
http://www.realfoodkosher.com
http://www.pubmed.gov

Step 7- No more added sugar, in any form: no honey, agave, or date sugar.

Here's why: Some sugar substitutes that are sweet, but made from chemicals (and some that are from natural sources) still make our brains and bodies think we have had sugar. This triggers cravings. Remember that sweets are treats, not to be indulged in daily, even if they are natural. I can easily eat a one pound box of dates in about 15 minutes. How about you?

You have progressed almost all the way through the Guide. **Steps 4 and 5** were the biggest challenges by far for most of you. This one should be a breeze. You are off the hamster wheel of sugar in its secret disguises.

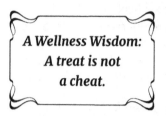

**A Wellness Wisdom:
A treat is not
a cheat.**

What I have found to be true for myself and for most of my coaching clients is that we slowly use less and less of the sweet natural substitutes until we use nothing in our coffee or tea. I rarely eat fruit, perhaps four times a year, only when I crave it. When I crave fruit I do not deny myself. I am truly listening to my body's needs. If I crave it I must need a vitamin, mineral, enzyme, or chemical from it that I am lacking. I went a year without a banana one time. Then one afternoon not too long ago, I saw bananas on the kitchen table and quietly but urgently ate three. My husband's eyes widened and he said, "Are you okay?" I replied, "Yes, I guess I needed a banana." Eating real food and eating clean for over five years has afforded me the ability to listen to my body very well. Free at last.

Buy the natural sugar alternatives Lakanto or XYLA on line or at health food stores. Lakanto is Chinese monk fruit dried and crystallized. It is used in Asia for lung issues, liver ailments, circulation, sore throats, and preventing a host of other illnesses. I like the golden brown variety of Lakanto. I buy Lakanto on the internet. Xyla is a natural white sugar alternative from the bark of the birch tree. I buy Xyla from a health food store. I use these natural sugar substitutes in my beverages and in marinades, dressings, sauces, and for baking.

When you want a treat, it is not a cheat. There is no self induced guilt here (and all guilt is truly self-induced). I believe in the 80/20 rule. That means if I eat clean and green 80 percent of the time I can party like a rock star 20 percent of the time. What you consistently practice 80 percent of the time shows up in your life 100 percent of the time. After years of clean eating my party choices aren't regularly gluten-filled, sugary chocolate cakes. The party looks more like a Manhattan cocktail and the following recipe. Enjoy this sugar free and grain free dessert recipe my daughter Sage (age 11 at the time) and I created:

CHOCOLATE BARK, FONDUE, AND TRUFFLE BASE

INGREDIENTS:

- 6 Tablespoons salted butter
- 1/4 cup Xyla or Lakanto (natural sweeteners)
- 2 Tablespoons coconut milk
- 1 4-ounce bar of 100% chocolate, broken into pieces (you may use raw chocolate if you want)
- Extra heavy whipping cream if you want less dark chocolate as the end result. Sometimes we will make dark milk chocolate, extra dark chocolate, and black chocolate truffle varieties in the same day.
- Optional Add-Ins: dried fruits, fruits, shredded coconut, cayenne or chili pepper, smoked paprika, cinnamon, nutmeg, pumpkin pie spice, vanilla, nuts, seeds, vegetables, dehydrated vegetables, etc.
- Mini cupcake paper liner

DIRECTIONS:

1. Put a small pan or small soup pot on medium heat.
2. Add the butter and sweetener to pot.
3. Stir until sweetener completely dissolves.
4. Add coconut milk and stir vigorously
5. Add chocolate pieces.
6. As the chocolate begins to melt, reduce heat to low and continue stirring until smooth.

7. Sometimes the chocolate is completely melted and mixed in, but has a grainy look within the smoothness, that is fine. It depends on the country of the chocolate's origin.

8. Once everything is done melting, you are ready to enjoy!

9. For fondue, leave the pot on the lowest simmer setting or on the table if the room is warm. Add extra heavy whipping cream to the pot if the desired result is less dark, experiment to your tastes.

10. Begin dipping your fruit or vegetables into the chocolaty goodness.

11. For adventurous types, try dipping broccoli or carrots into the fondue!

12. For truffles, use a teaspoon and drop a teaspoon or more of the chocolate into mini candy molds or mini cupcake liners.

13. Press shredded coconut, nuts, or dried fruits on top.

14. Place in freezer at least one hour. Makes 18 truffles.

15. For bark, line a cookie sheet with parchment paper.

16. Place nuts, seeds, or dried fruits on paper, then pour chocolate on top evenly covering the goodies.

17. Freeze at least an hour. Enjoy.

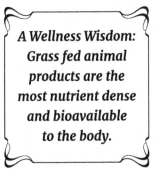

A Wellness Wisdom: Grass fed animal products are the most nutrient dense and bioavailable to the body.

Step 8- Purchase raw dairy and pasture-raised eggs if you regularly consume dairy and eggs. Pasture-raised eggs are eggs from chickens who aren't fed grains, and are free to roam about to eat bugs, worms, fruits, grasses, and vegetables.

Here's why: Raw dairy and 100% pasture-raised eggs may not cause the same reaction to the body as products from grain fed animals. If you are sensitive to dairy and grains I suggest trying baby steps and tread lightly with this one. On an empty stomach try one taste of one product that is the highest quality and not factory farmed, make sure that they are 100% grass fed dairy and unpasteurized. If eggs, make certain they are not fed grains and that they are 100% pastured, and not fed hormones and antibiotics. My own experience is that I no longer suffer from constipation or rashes when I eat raw milk, cream, and cheeses. The pastured eggs just taste better, although I never had any sensitivity to eggs.

Remember, if you consume animal products, you eat what the animal ate. If an animal does not have grains in its natural diet and we give it grains, antibiotics, and growth hormones, it may suffer allergies, bloating, obesity, stress, illness, etc. When we eat an animal, its milk, or its offspring, we may literally eat the stress and illness, or suffer the resulting effects from the hormones and medicines the farmers feed them. They suffer, we suffer. They stress, we stress. They get fat, we get fat. They are ill, we are ill. Everything is connected.

I know pastured eggs are more expensive than regularly produced eggs. I know raw milk and cheeses are costly when compared to pasteurized, processed cheeses. You have just given up all grains, fruits, and sugars. You no longer have processed foods in your cupboards. There are no sodas, breads, pies, cakes cookies, cereal, pasta, crackers, chips, corn chips, tortillas, ice cream, or pizzas in the house. Cereal is upwards of $5.00 a box. With the money you have been saving throughout the steps thus far, you may afford a higher quality food supply or go on a higher quality vacation.

Step 9- Give up beans and legumes.

Here's why: Beans and legumes are high starch and must be soaked overnight and then cooked to release the gaseous property. They have a hard endosperm covering which must be broken down in order to be absorbed by the body. For years the media has promoted beans as high protein, but most beans and legumes have about 30% protein. Mostly beans are carbohydrates, which raises blood sugar. I tend to steer clear of them for my tummy's sake.

When I crave a bean-like texture I eat roasted chestnuts, already shelled. They are so delicious and nutritious. Lucky for me, they are readily available in stores in Northern California.

In all of the steps, pay particular attention to how you feel rather than how you look. Sometimes flu and cold symptoms, headaches, and general fatigue may plague you. You may suffer acne or a rash for a little while. These are symptoms of the body detoxifying and getting used to the cleaner fuel you are providing it with. Fear not, and keep moving forward with the process. Moving toward superior health can spur us on to our true self. Just think about how clear, attentive, helpful, and generous you can be towards others you love after you have taken care of your own essential biochemical needs. It's not about the food, although your relationship with food tends to become healthier overall. It's about a *Happy, Healthy, You.*

This guide is an example of methodical action. You can use this example for any goal in mind. Work at a pace where you can just keep going. Make it a survival pace at first. When we first attempt things unfamiliar to us, they seem impossible. Take one step. Perfect that one step. Own it. The boundaries and limits have just been moved a bit farther past what you formerly thought was doable.

Then take the second step. Before you know it you are leaping ahead in your life in all facets because you took the first step and didn't give up.

After you have completed **Superior Self's Guide to Wellness from Within** on your own terms and on your own time frame, your palate will change. You will see food as fuel. Real food will taste enhanced and will be more delicious than ever. Your internal self will shift as well. You will be emotionally more even because there will be none of those chemical additives and preservatives messing with your pleasure hormones in the brain.

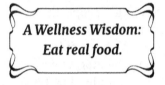

A Wellness Wisdom:
Eat real food.

Most psychiatric patients are also dealing with digestive disorders.[4] There is a link between mental illness symptoms and the intestinal bacteria being out of balance. When we have a toxic intestine, there are weak walls. The toxic bacteria can permeate (get through) the walls. The toxic bacteria are then carried throughout the entire body by the blood. This may create a river of mental and physiological problems. We may feel out of sorts, physically ill, and mentally stuck. Depression, a sense of being overwhelmed, and a host of other disorders may prevail, keeping us paralyzed. So, how can we heal and move forward? Nourishing ourselves with a variety of real, whole foods is a great start. Replanting the intestines with fermented foods that contain probiotics adds another layer of healing. Consuming naturally raw, fermented foods like raw sauerkraut, plain Greek yogurt, and kefir are a good place to begin. They add good bacteria back into the body and reduce levels of toxicity, while building immunity. A dietary overhaul is part of a holistic approach to healing, in body and in mind.

"Let food be thy medicine and medicine be thy food."
—Hippocrates

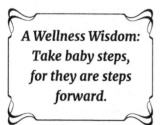

A Wellness Wisdom:
Take baby steps,
for they are steps
forward.

We can improve our lives, no matter what our current circumstances are. I know this sounds hard to believe, especially when we feel like we have been through hell, but it is the absolute truth.

It may take a billion baby steps, but baby steps are steps, after all! Tiny improvements are positive affirmations of what we humans are capable of overcoming.

How we think about ourselves affects how other people think about us. What we think about, we bring about. I have heard this phrase in so many ways and from so many people, but it didn't touch my life personally until I heard it from my mentor, Colin F. Watson, my health and life coach. He came into my life while I was working on my own mid-life wellness goals, when I felt stuck.

Colin said the self-loathing we exude when we pass a mirror, glance at our reflection, and mentally criticize ourselves is the reason why our fat loss and fitness goals may not be realized. We may work out and eat well, but negative internal dialogue, when combined with daily stress, lack of sleep, and modern anxieties acts like a dam in the waterfall. We then may cheat on our actions related to our other life goals because, "Who are we kidding anyway? We failed so many times before."

The inner critic pops into our heads all the time, every day. It is natural to have this visitor. *It's just not the truth.* Somehow we got frozen. We can also get unfrozen. With self-love and making sure we take care of our heart first, we can cure the internal self-loathing. We can feel fully awesome and capable of doing anything again.

I want to tell you a story about self-love silencing the inner critic, and instead saying *thank you,* all day long.

Graces's Story: no whining or complaining despite cancer

Grace and Chuy were regulars at my hotel restaurant. They were in their seventies and loved to sit next to each other instead of across from each other while eating. Chuy would squish himself into the tiny booth for two, next to Grace, practically sitting on his wife's knee. One evening while enjoying dinner, he explained why. "I have a short umbilical cord connecting me to my wife," he lovingly explained, as he gestured from his belly towards his wife's, pointing with his long elegant fingers.

A few minutes later I brought them their half-chicken dinner to share. Chuy reluctantly moved across the table to his own single seat to eat dinner, knowing full well that by dessert he would be sitting next to Grace and sharing a small dessert that required no sharp knives nor hot cast iron skillets.

"Why do you have such a short umbilical cord?" I asked.

"We met when we were fifteen years old. We have been together ever since. About five years ago, Grace got cancer. Through her cancer treatments, I still had to work [Chuy works for a fine chocolate company]. I went with Grace to chemotherapy when I could, but it was after each treatment that we had our healing time together. I would tell her to bring it in, meaning come and hold me, tummy to tummy."

Whatever pain, nausea, fear, worry, uncertainty, and negative thoughts Grace experienced dissipated. Even now, they have *bring it in* moments daily, and Grace is celebrating five years cancer free. The umbilical cord expression makes sense to me now.

Grace further explained, "I was always a praying individual with a good attitude. I listened to my body very well. I stayed busy, but if I needed rest, I rested. I didn't pray to God to heal me from cancer. I prayed to God in gratitude. I said thanks for the person who mopped the floor to make my chemotherapy room sanitary and safe. I prayed thank you to God for creating a warm and loving environment for my treatments. I prayed a prayer of gratitude for the nurses choosing a career path they love and are passionate about. I prayed a prayer of thanks for the doctors to do their jobs well and with compassion. I prayed that God would bestow comfort and courage to the mothers in the neighboring rooms who were caring for their children here with chemotherapy, yet also neglecting their other children at home because of their situation."

Grace didn't ask or beg for her cancer to be healed. She didn't have a death wish, she told me. Grace had days full of thankfulness, with a wide smile and pep in her step. She didn't feel like God was punishing her for eating junk food during her early years. She just was not ready for the pity party. She was not one to cry and ask over and over again, "Why me?" Not that the question isn't valid, but it does not move one forward. Grace wanted to move forward and wanted to find the small steps toward healing through grace, literally and figuratively. She really lived up to her name. Grace created a *Happy, Healthy You.*

A Mindfulness Moment:
I'm not perfect.
I'm beautiful.

Self doubt has a crippling effect on everything we do. It can seep into our bones like arthritis, little bit by little bit. At first, we can take an aspirin or ibuprofen to stave it off, but as it takes over our body, we give in to it. No. I say, no. Then, after the positive work, using the tools throughout this book and after we shift, when we pass a mirror or store window, and notice our reflection, we can smile, nod, and say in our heads, "Hello, fabulous!".

An Invitation: less than perfect

Breaking someone down with tough love doesn't always make them stronger. Sometimes it just breaks them down. Write down three things that you hold in your mind and body that tell you that you aren't good enough.

Write down the age that you first felt this way. Put the paper into the *Negative Thought Pot*. Set it on fire and watch it burn to ashes. Boom! Gone. Smile.

An Invitation: mirror positivity and grace

Go stand directly in front of a mirror. Smile at yourself. Observe your smile, your teeth, and your twinkling eyes. Say to yourself out loud, but quietly, "Thank you for all the miraculous things you do for me every day. I love and respect you."

Do this again tomorrow, and the day after...

We tend to generalize about ourselves in terms of self-judgment, just as much as we generalize about others. I feel this is dangerous because we are constantly changing and evolving as humans. What was true about me a week ago, or even a moment ago, may not necessarily be true right now.

When we look at the facts and our beliefs, we can see how one influences the other. For example, my legs are long. Physically, I will not be able to have my eyebrows touch my toes when stretching in the "eyes to toes" yoga pose. But if I keep telling myself that one day I will do it, I will make the effort to stretch deeper and deeper into the pose and go further than I ever have before. After all, it is the goal and the name of the pose. My belief changed the length of the stretch over time. Never say never.

Our perceptions and others' perceptions of the facts can influence us in positive ways, even when they are completely false! When I saw Oprah complete her first marathon at age forty, I decided right then and there that when I turned forty, I would be mature enough, and have enough mental strength, endurance, and power to run a marathon. So, a day or so before my fortieth birthday I ran and completed my first marathon. (Since then, I have completed sixteen marathons.)

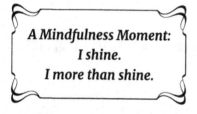

A Mindfulness Moment:
I shine.
I more than shine.

My daughter was a toddler at the time. When she saw the crowd, music, balloons, and fanfare as they announced my name crossing the finish line, she thought I won the marathon, taking first place. I had a medal, tee shirt, and food as gifts too. Her believing I won made it so in her world. The facts and the beliefs worked together in assisting me in accomplishing my goals. They are powerful tools. Since then, every time I get near the end of a race, when I hear my name, see the balloons, and music is blaring, I feel like I have won. I get emotional and teary eyed. I feel immensely grateful for my heart, arms, legs, and life. Thanks, Oprah.

Just recognizing that beginning spot, the root of our rut, is awareness. It is an opening of the exit door with the exit light illuminated. Push the exit door open further and step on through. You *are* good enough. You are *more* than good enough. You *shine*. You *more* than shine. If nobody shared that with you before, allow me to do that now. You *are* the illumination that lights up your own universe, as well as the lives of others. Do not rely on others to tell you so. Sometimes, ancient, hidden memories can be triggered by something seemingly unrelated to them in our current life. When the floodgate of recollections opens up, try not to suppress them. They are a gift to you now, so that you may begin to deal with them, learn from them, and heal from them. Facing our difficulties *does* make us stronger.

I believe in the power of humans to sparkle, glitter, shine, spread love, and exude positive thoughts. This is despite the crises that have happened to us in our past. I witness the sparkle every day in the very busy hotel restaurant where I work. Strangers touch my heart with simple gestures, inspirational stories, and wisdom-filled memories shared. I watch as disharmony shifts into harmony amongst families on their vacations to San Francisco. I am a fly on the wall at anniversaries, weddings, and the breathtaking, "Will you marry me?" Conversations with my guests give me continued hope of conquering our demons, our pasts, and what paralyzes us.

When we do these written and active exercises, we can have the inside out approach to healing. We can heal from the negative self-talk and from the childhood beliefs of being *less than*. We can get to the root of the rut

Fuel, Focus, Foundation

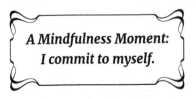

A Mindfulness Moment: I commit to myself.

Food as **fuel** is an important viewpoint as we end this chapter. If you didn't have to think about what you are going to eat for breakfast, lunch and dinner anymore and you weren't ruled by fake foods, food would be just fuel, like gas in the fuel tank of your car. If you had food freedom, would you find other sorts of emotional freedom? What bonds would you break free from?

Food as **focus** is an important viewpoint as we end this chapter. If you could focus on your other goals in life once you attained food freedom, what would they be? What unique imprint would you impress upon the earth? What would your legacy be?

Food as **foundation** is an important viewpoint as we end this chapter. Are you a stronger human being now that you know the interconnectedness of the intake of substances from the earth and the relationship between the foods we eat, the beliefs we have, our attitude, and our past experiences?

Food as **fuel**, **focus**, and **foundation** work together in supporting a *Happy, Healthy You.*

Chapter Two

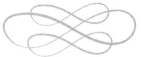

What Is Trauma Anyway? Trauma vs. Drama

When a person experiences intense emotional, psychological, or physical injury, one is said to have experienced trauma. The impact of unprocessed trauma, whether it is temporary or permanent, can keep one from fully living. One may feel as if living in an alternate reality for a while; *here*, but not fully here. One may be able to get through the day and competently complete daily responsibilities (work, cooking, cleaning, childrearing, spousal duties, etc.), but underneath the surface, a tornado of emotional turmoil may be whirling.

There is this deep unexplainable experience that occurs alongside of the injury. There is no logic involved. It is darkness. Initially, there's no seeing through it. In the process of healing, when we get to the other side of the darkness, it makes no sense either, at first. It seems like the darkness has lifted though, and that is enough.

"Stars can't shine without darkness."
—Unknown

We are entitled to miracles and lightness of being every day, but we tend to block them, even if we have not suffered much. I encourage you to change these expectations. *Expect good things to happen.* How? How do we do that when we have suffered tragedy, crises, and severe pain that no one really understands? Keep reading, my friends. Trust the process.

My Story: everyday miracles: teasing the rainbow out from the clouds

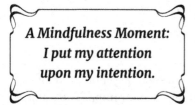

A Mindfulness Moment: I put my attention upon my intention.

My teenage son and I were driving to the famous Winchester Mystery Mansion for my 51st birthday. I had never been there before and the history of the stories surrounding the mansion was fascinating. Halloween was the next day so the event was a candlelight tour at night. The clouds were gray and it looked like rain. As we drove 45 minutes to San Jose from San Francisco, I saw the sunshine peeping at me from my rear view mirror. "All right, Golden," I said. "Let's bring a rainbow out for my birthday." I rubbed my thumb against my first two fingers of my right hand in a gesture meaning *money*. In my case, I was teasing out a rainbow, thinking, "Come on, come on, lucky rainbow, lucky me." Wouldn't you know it, less than 10 minutes into my efforts a beautiful double rainbow appeared to the left side of the freeway? Was it a miracle? Am I a conjurer of rainbows? Or was it a result of me placing my *attention* upon my *intention*?

"The way I see it, if you want the rainbow, you gotta put up with the rain."
—Dolly Parton, singer and actor

Other examples of everyday miracles:

- Parking angels who open up a spot right in front of the venue you are going to.

- Parking meters with money and time left inside.

- Parking meters that are broken and someone taped a sturdy sign with permanent marker to it.

- A stranger smiling at you for no reason and no hidden agenda.

- Having just enough cream left in the refrigerator for my coffee.

- Checking off everything on the to-do list and still having time to exercise and meditate before cooking and cleaning.

- Seeing a ball bounce into your neighborhood street and instinctively knowing a child will follow, so you just put your emergency blinkers on and wait patiently, avoiding disaster, and instead creating a miracle.

An Invitation: everyday miracles - expect good things to happen

Make a short list of *lucky* events that happen to you as they occur. Make a conscious effort to view them as everyday miracles even though the concept may not be in your wheelhouse. "Find a penny, pick it up. All day long you'll have good luck." I chanted this as a kid and taught my kids this thank you ritual when finding coins on the sidewalk or street. Now, as teens, my kids still chant it when they see a coin on the ground and pick it up. The more you list the small everyday miracles, the more you will observe and be expecting them. More tiny miracles or lucky events will happen.

How does this relate to trauma? It is all energy, and the positive things you expect and put out will help in the healing process from trauma as well.

Psychological trauma is when a person suffers deeply, perhaps from horrifying events, such as continued physical abuse, continued emotional abuse, or a terrorist attack. Psychological trauma is long lasting and can be quite overwhelming to an individual. It may lead to long term anxiety, distress and stress.[5]

Not all traumatic events lead to psychological trauma. If we are healthy human beings, have a support system in place, have a strong family and community foundation, and generally feel loved unconditionally, we can recover well, and relatively rapidly.

If we are unhealthy or suffer repeated abuse, our psychological and physical body reacts poorly afterward, and we cannot cope as easily. When the body reacts poorly, we see physiological effects from trauma. Our biological markers may be poor, and can be identified by taking physicals and blood tests.

When we suffer deeply, we may require extra assistance in order to recover and thrive. It may take a long time to heal, but we *can* heal.

Initially after the traumatic event, we generally cope in a few common ways:

1. We may zone out; this is called dissociation.

2. We may excite the fear centers of the brain, thus affecting general memory. The fear centers may have us feeling anxious all the time, even during mild, everyday activities.

3. We may have flashbacks to the incident, either in our waking visual memory, or in auditory memory. Flashbacks also can come as nightmares when we are sleeping.[6]

My Story: burn victim

My own experience with trauma took place when I was the victim of a hot water travel cup explosion.

I was heading by car on the freeway towards my daughter's summer day camp for pickup. I went to take a sip of hot water out of my travel mug. The inner factory seal exploded upwards, and all of the contents cascaded onto my body.

I immediately thought of fire ants. The burning was so intense, for a few seconds I didn't realize that fire ants were not the cause of the heat sensation. I started deep yoga breathing in order to not have an accident on the freeway.

When I finally put cool water on my burns, I was at the closest gas station. I sat on the ground next to the building with the water flowing on my body from an outdoor spigot. I sat there in a daze with all of my clothes on. I was silent, I didn't cry or scream, but I disappeared for a few minutes. I zoned out immediately (dissociation).

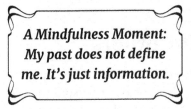

A Mindfulness Moment: My past does not define me. It's just information.

For a year or more afterwards, I had nightmares and flashbacks of the incident. I burst into night sweats often during the nightmares, and experienced rapid heart palpitations. My husband woke me up from a deep sleep often, telling me that I was crying in my sleep. My flashbacks varied in intensity, length of time and the emotions accompanying them. Even to this day, every time I pass that particular gas station, the whole horrid accident reoccurs in my mind. My heart races, I begin to perspire, and I pray a prayer of grace. It could have been way worse. This is a clear example of physiological trauma symptoms, and how they can continue long after the physical wounds have healed.

I sometimes experienced other stress related symptoms resulting from the incident, like sleepless nights and jumpiness around tea kettles (and pots with boiling water in them). When these tensions rose up inside of me, I made a conscious decision toward a more positive end. I used the time and nervous energy to research all things spiritual and scientific related to my area of interest, wellness though nutrition. I worked on my blog and newsletters. I chose not to dwell in the misery of my past and the *what ifs*. I consciously chose to use the energy as a springboard upwards in my humanity, even as I recalled the tragedy. I chose to become my superior self.

Sometimes helping others is a tool we can use to stop dwelling and take the focus off of ourselves. No more *poor me*. I began coaching others on wellness almost immediately after the burn incident. I didn't realize at the time, that this was my coping mechanism. In helping others become healthier and more energetic, I was healing myself too. For me, this was a way out of my sadness, my feelings of being a helpless victim, and a break from the repeated internal question, "Why me?"

An Invitation: mentor others

We all have strengths and expertise in some area. Whatever your area of passion is, choose to assist another person or persons in that area. Be open to others asking for your help. Do not deny your authority. When stepping outside of ourselves and helping others, we confirm what we already know. It is greatly satisfying to help other people grow in something.

When mentoring others, practice patience. Allow the mentee to see errors being made. The learner needs to see our mistakes, faults, and errors. Remember, the word *mentor* is not the same word as the word *tormentor*. There is no pressure here to be a perfectionist. Show others how growth can be garnished from errors. Problems can be a source of strength if we don't hide it from others. *Nobody's perfect. Everybody's beautiful.*

"Reach out and touch somebody's hand. Make this a better place, if you can."
—Nickolas Ashford and Valerie Simpson

The Difference Between Trauma and Drama

In today's world we live in such a media driven, sensationalist society that we are numbed to the differences between trauma and drama. Perhaps these illustrations may clear things up.

- **Drama** may be when you just suffered a break up with your boyfriend whom you have been seeing for two months.

- **Drama** may be if my sister-in-law is changing her gender through surgery and becoming her most authentic self, free at last (traumatic for her, but not for the general public).

- **Drama** may be when I'm stuck in traffic, my phone died, I cannot pick up my child at school on time, I do not have a backup plan, and she is waiting in the principal's office for me, wondering and worrying about where I am.

These are everyday life dramas and sensational dramas that we blow up out of proportion. We tend to think about and express them as traumatic events. They are not.

- **Trauma** may be when you are giving birth to your first born, she is still born, and you almost die from complications in the labor and delivery room.

- **Trauma** may be watching your loved one perish in an apartment fire, from the street, when you have just been saved by firefighters, and they are desperately trying to get your other family members out before the building crumbles to the ground. You are speaking to your betrothed by cell phone, saying final words of love and devotion.

- **Trauma** may be walking down the street after getting off of the bus in the early evening, and being dragged away, beaten, raped, and left for dead in plain view of a busy gas station.

I sincerely hope these examples clarify the differences between trauma and drama. This book seeks to assist in rising up from trauma and drama. The stories and exercises may be read in any order and practiced for any length of time. The main point for me is to share with you that in order to get anywhere, we have to start somewhere. Why not here? Why not now?

Asking for Help is Not a Sign of Weakness

Being a mentor is a wonderful way to heal ourselves while helping others, but on the other hand, do not be afraid to admit to being in a state of lack. It is perfectly okay to ask for help too. Personally, I think it is imperative to seek out those who know more than we do during the quest for healing and growth, in any and every area of life.

Do you want to learn how to crochet? Ask a master crochet artist or someone who teaches it at a local arts center. Do you want to run a marathon? Ask someone who has run one or more some questions. Get books on marathons from the library, subscribe to a running magazine, listen to professional runners speak about marathons on a podcast, join a running club, etc. Make a plan and stick to it.

We are not weak if we ask for help. Usually someone who really knows their subject will be flattered that you asked them. We are making a strong, bold move in recognizing our limitations. We may receive a myriad of benefits by picking the brain, so to speak, of someone else who is at the top of their game and is willing to share.

In order to have some sort of relief from our past or current problems, it may be helpful to reach outward at the same time that we are reaching inward. Seek out books, workshops, social workers, counselors, psychologists, therapists, etc. Build a community of support that will be a strong foundation. Reach out to a religious leader or a counseling group. Find a coach. We *will* grow, heal, and thrive as humans when we ask for help, and receive it. We must, however, commit to the process. We have the *right* to feel connected again. We have the *right* to feel whole again. We *will* have the power to feel productive in society again, if we reach out and say, "Will you help me?".

⸕⸎⸕

Anger, frustration, pride: they all get in the way sometimes, even in the absence of a major trauma. Our sense of freedom, hope, and future possibility may be compromised during our lives, especially after abuses.

We like to hold off on being happy, anyway. Why? Even if we don't have life-altering trauma, we seek it out by watching others. We are voyeurs. I think it is because we see the media as a gauge of ourselves. Scandals, gossip, and celebrity drama are so exciting, and they get ratings too. This happens at work and in the family dynamics as well. Who doesn't gossip at work or at the family reunion BBQ?

We do have the choice, however, to turn this around. Use problems within this life as opportunities for growth. We can also minimize the small challenges instead of blowing every little thing out of proportion. (You know exactly what I'm talking about.) We can turn lemons into lemonade and sour apples into cider. Drink the goodness, and discard the rest when you can. Weed out the non-important stuff from our path, so we can be steadier in our life's mission.

⟡

Juliette's Story: knowing how to ask for help

Juliette really took to baking from an early age. Her parents met as teenagers working in a small, family owned coffee house in Rehoboth Beach, Delaware.

During high school, they worked part time in the coffee house, learning how to make all of the handmade baked goods from scratch.

They married soon after college, and had Juliette a year or so later. The owners of the coffee house retired, and they sold the business to Juliette's parents. Her family clearly loved the community, as well as the baking environment.

As a toddler, Juliette would sit on the large wood table where they rolled out dough, and make her own shapes, add flavors, and generally make messes. The sights, sounds, and smells of the coffee house and bakery intrigued the toddler, as all of her senses were engaged. As she got older, Juliette became a passionate baker, experimenting with lavender, chili, squid ink, and other non-traditional flavor profiles and ingredients.

This was her strong and loving childhood foundation. The family unit was unconditionally there for her, and so was the tight-knit community. The sights, sounds, and smells of the café, its patrons, baked goods, music, and coffee defined *home*. The café was her safe space, and was a constant comfort.

During her first year in college, Juliette ran into some trouble with credit card hackers. Somehow they stole her identity twice in six months, and took her bank accounts, her school scholarship fund, and her social security number. After the initial freak-out of screaming and crying, Juliette did what she knew best. She made a beeline to the coffee house. Baking was her coping mechanism. After baking up a storm, Juliette was able to calm down and call the bank and the social security office, and then handle other tasks that needed to be dealt with.

She had a great support system. Juliette knew who she could call upon for help. Baking was her way of handling the dramatic situation both practically and emotionally. I say practically because it allowed her to be able to carry out the practical steps in order to solve the problem in a peaceful manner.

Juliette's story is a reminder for us of the difference between a dramatic event and a traumatic event. Perhaps if she was a child of teenaged parents who had been given up for foster care, or worse, an abused child of drug addicts, she would not have had the strong foundation and safe space to deal with the challenge.

What does one do if one is living in a less than ideal environment and something crappy like that happens? Who can one ask for help? How do we know who we can trust? There are many things one can do, and sometimes just ten seconds of deep breathing can calm us down enough to think of the *one* person who can be called upon for help.

Building a community of support happens randomly sometimes. Communication creates connection, which creates community. When a café opened up recently with fresh, local, and gluten free options, I walked in and ordered from the coffee barista. Now I see the staff almost daily and communicate regularly with them about the kids, politics, art, or life in general. The few folks who come to the café at the same time I do for coffee have a rhythm going.

We are having repeated communication and building a thread. The thread is now a connection. I look forward to seeing the baristas and the other patrons for small talk or a deep conversation. The staff always makes my cappuccino extra hot without me asking because they know that's just how I like it. They are my café family in my neighborhood. We have a connection and are building a community. I trust them and know I can go to them for certain emergencies.

Daily Foundation: Build Your Happy, Healthy Day from the Ground Up

Just like Juliette had a strong life foundation, we can also affirm our daily activities with a positive foundation, no matter what our personal background. We have the gift of choice every day. If we set up our day with a non-dramatic foundation, our day is set up well.

Personally, I wake up each day, stretch, make my coffee, drink water, take my vitamins, and play peaceful piano music on the stereo or phone. I pray a silent gratitude prayer, and smile at myself as I brush my teeth. Good morning world! If I set my day up with a positive vibe, a foundation of *yes*, I'm pretty certain the rest of my day will follow suit.

The opposite is also true. If I scowl and shout expletives, rush, and make my coffee too weak, my foundation for the day is also weak. I will most likely have a crappy, weak day, fraught with negatives. I will have a slowly downward spiraling day.

The key word in the above paragraph is *rush*. Rushing solves no problems and usually causes dramatic events, so it is a poor foundation. You will do yourself and the world a favor by giving yourself a do-over. Take ten seconds to stop the insanity. Inhale and exhale slowly, to regroup. Slow down. You will arrive *there* anyway, just ten seconds later. This is your life, remember? Don't you deserve to be happy in it, today, now? Set yourself up for success with a positive daily foundation.

Life is like the day to day set up too. If one has a strong, positive upbringing with loving parents and an unconditional support system in place, we see the likelihood of a strong life. Parents have the task of guiding their children well, hugging and kissing often, and modeling positive behavior. Parenting well is a huge responsibility and privilege. Be aware, however, that the set up is not always a prescription set in stone. (I am not living in a fairy tale.) Life does throw us curve balls. How we react is based upon our foundation, though. Sometimes it is based on how we have healed *after* a rough foundation.

"A setback is a setup for a comeback."
—Douglass Fitch, pastor, author

Amen.

Creating, Planting, and Watering the Seeds of Foundation

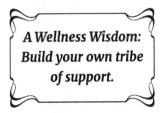

A Wellness Wisdom:
Build your own tribe
of support.

As in Chapter 1, here again we see the word foundation being used with intention. Sometimes we are not born with a strong family foundation, so we must create, plant, and water our own seeds of foundation. In Chapter 1, food was the foundation. Here we see the foundation being the strength of a support system, either from parents or a community, a strong instillation of self esteem, and if the $#!+ hits the fan, knowing it is okay to ask for help. At the end of the winding, bumpy road there can be a *Happy, Healthy You.*

Chapter Three

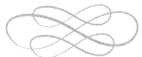

Sexual Trauma ~ You Can Overcome Anything

The title of this chapter alone may have some readers skipping over it. Perhaps some readers are squirming. If it does not apply to you personally, that's okay. You can still learn lessons here. Must one be totally screwed up in order to recover well and thoroughly from a bad experience? No. How we react and respond to a less than ideal situation may be an *aha* moment. If we learn from others' personal triumphs, those may hold value for us as well. Warning: this chapter may trigger memories and hidden experiences you may not have even remembered before reading this chapter. Breathe and hold yourself in the utmost place of self-care and love. If I am speaking directly to you, reach out to family or someone in the helping profession.

Most sexual trauma begins in childhood, and mostly to females. How a girl reacts to the abuse affects her entire development. She may develop personality changes, disorders, and lifestyle choices that are less than ideal or healthy.[7]

A few common, long term reactions seen in victims of sexual trauma are:

- Using drugs and alcohol

- Acting out sexually

- Eating too much or too little

- Cutting or hurting oneself

- Depression/Anxiety/Withdrawal

- Seeking therapy services

Sexual harassment, assault, abuse, or molestation can make people feel worthless, not worthy. Sometimes it can keep one from feeling worthy of love. It is easy to fill that void with other things, like food, alcohol, drugs, or obsessive habits. It is easy to create emotional obstacles.

Anastasia's Story: childhood sexual molestation

Anastasia was molested by adults in her family from an early age of seven, and the abuse lasted through her twelfth birthday.

She was unaware during the entire time, that she could have said the word NO. As a child of seven years old, what was running through Ana's mind was that she would be spanked if she said no. They were much bigger and stronger. Or even worse, she imagined they might tell on *her*, to her parents, and might twist things around to make her folks believe that she had approached the males, instead of the truth.

Somehow, Anastasia felt it might have truly been all her fault. She was a big hugger and kisser her whole life. She loved being babied, and adored being the center of attention at the large family parties. She received so much love and attention, that when things went awry, Ana didn't want to taint the fun times and close positive family relationships by telling her parents the negative activities that were going on, right under their noses.

Anastasia felt ashamed, embarrassed, and bad. She told herself she was a bad little girl. Ana did not have the courage to tell *anyone* older whom she trusted. She was afraid to ask for help *or* to make it stop on her own.

Anastasia developed a variety of defense mechanisms, the most visible being eating to stifle the pain and shame. Eating was also her tool to make herself less attractive, perhaps to make the abuse stop in a passive manner. It didn't, for a long time.

Ana ate herself into oblivion, consuming so many pastries and bowls of ice cream that the hours afterwards were spent in a "food coma." People joke about the term, but it was an honest and real way for her to escape.

Eventually she believed that she was pregnant because she was so fat, and she held her weight in her tummy area. Anastasia was too young to really understand how babies were made. In her innocent mind, fat equaled pregnant. Mentally, it was a totally separate thing from what she was experiencing with the older male relatives.

To deal with the "pregnancy," Anastasia punched herself in the stomach daily in order to attempt to get rid of the nonexistent baby. She was black and blue and sore from the self-inflicted beatings in the corner of her lavender wallpapered bedroom. In the seven year old's mind, fat equaled pregnant, and bad things happening *to her* equaled that *she was* a bad little girl.

The eating thing became a double edged sword. When Anastasia ate more than one helping at meals, it was considered a compliment to her immigrant mama, who prided herself on being a gourmet cook. The more Ana ate, the more her mother looked upon her daughter as a good and perfect little girl. In little Ana's head, it became a way to bond even more closely to her mother, as well as a chance to become unattractive to her abusers.

> **The definition of sexual abuse is any unwanted sexual contact that is performed by someone older or more powerful than the victim.**

As she grew to be an obese child of ten years old, Anastasia developed the belief that the sexual abuse was the only way she could get outside attention, especially from the opposite sex, because fat people are usually ignored or made fun of. Attention of any kind was a desirable thing (or so she thought). She saw how women flocked to the male abusers at church and at church picnics. Ana was getting fatter and fatter, yet they still came around. Part of her subconscious mind rationalized that if she was obese, and they still wanted her, she must have value. Another part of her desperately wanted them to stop. Ana was deeply conflicted and confused.

Ana felt like she was a secret family disgrace. On the surface, she was all straight A's and church choir soloist, the perfect student and daughter. Underneath, however, something else was brewing.

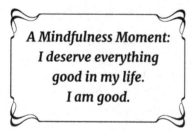

A Mindfulness Moment:
I deserve everything
good in my life.
I am good.

It wasn't until her first holy communion at around age twelve, that Anastasia had an epiphany. The ceremony resonated within her seat of power, her soul and heart. After the ceremony, there was a huge party at her parents' home. Once again, Ana was cornered by the male relatives upstairs while the festivities were going on outside. She calmly and clearly stated, "No. We are done. Go find yourselves, get therapy, and get healed. God doesn't like ugly, and you both have been ugly in so many ways. Leave me alone!" That was the end of the abuse.

Anastasia realized for the first time that she had the power to say no. She had an *aha* moment. She never told her parents and she never asked the male relatives to apologize. As an adult, Anastasia told her mama after she was married with children. Her mama was shocked and sorry, of course. Had her mother known, she would have done anything to help her baby heal from the pain and suffering.

During the abusive years, Anastasia rationalized every move the abusers made by telling herself that is how people learn about sex. Better with people she *knew* than with strangers...

After Anastasia finally said no, she was able to conquer the pounds of pain, mentally and physically. Then, another turn of events took place; Ana began throwing up her meals with regularity. She became bulimic. During the time she stopped punching herself in the stomach, she punished herself with constant self monitoring and self-judgment. The balance was lost, even as she healed from the men abusing her. She kept food diaries, another way of being in control of something. Bulimia and constantly monitoring her food intake were ways of keeping boys and men away. She was too *busy* getting fat or thin or *something, anything* to keep away from males.

Anastasia came to me as an adult in her fifties. We had deep heart to heart talks, and we used the *Negative Thought Pot* with regularity. After months of practice with the pot, and practicing loving herself deeply, Ana was able to free herself from the control issues, the self abuse, and the discomfort of her past. Anastasia began lifting weights for the first time at the gym, and her inner and outer strengths grew in a parallel rhythm.

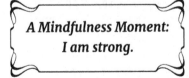

**A Mindfulness Moment:
I am strong.**

She became a strong and powerful weight lifter, and even joined in competitions. Her story and confidence are an inspiration to many. Now she is not afraid to share her story, anywhere, anytime. When Anastasia placed the blame where it belonged, she could move on once and for all.

During our time together, we engaged in role play. I, of course, had to play the roles of her perpetrators. Anastasia told me what she really thought of me (the abusers). She cried, she screamed, and she gave herself the freedom to finally let go.

"Unfortunately, sometimes people don't hear you until you scream."
—Stefanie Powers, actor

An Invitation: write nasty people off

Think of the people who have done you wrong. Sometimes it is not your fault and they are *not* reacting to your mean actions toward them. They are nasty because nasty things have been showed to them as *normal behavior*.

Role play with someone you trust, someone who can role play well in acting nasty towards you in an exercise like this one. Tell them off, BIG TIME. Tell them it is not okay, and why. Tell them why you deserve love and light, moments of laughter and friendship, or any kind of respectful relationship. Tell them goodbye if you need to. Allow yourself the freedom that goes along with saying *no*, and give yourself the freedom of letting go of unacceptable activities.

This does not only have to be an exercise related specifically to sexual abuses. Feel free to pull it out of the wellness toolkit at any time.

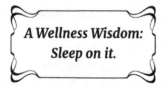

A Wellness Wisdom:
Sleep on it.

After this exercise, perhaps you will be ready to *tell off* the actual nasty person or persons the next time you are in their presence. Maybe now you will seek them out for this particular intended task. Are you ready?

Ok, so that was a heavy and exhausting exercise. Now what? *Rest.*
Rest in the space that comes with peace. We need peace in that
spongy, in-between phase before going on to build what we think is
acceptable, what is okay, and what is welcoming in our lives.

One day I was in yoga class; at the end of class we have a two minute
savasana, which is a quiet and silent rest on the floor, lying on our
backs, facing up. I closed my eyes and thought, "I want to rest in
peace, before I *rest in peace.*"In my head, I decided a pure and
disconnected moment out of my body would be amazing. I wanted
to feel what leaving my body would be like before I really died, left
my body, and rested in peace permanently. I read about people who
meditate deeply enough to leave their physical selves with silver
thread connecting them. That would be nice to do.

Sacred Living Through Everyday Actions

When we are rested, truly rested after the hard work done above, we
can then meander about in our heads with what we are ready to do
in our lives and what we are willing to go after, accept or not accept
now. I say build sacred living through every day actions. Create daily
rituals that make gratitude a part of the action.

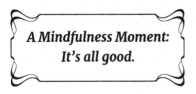

A Mindfulness Moment:
It's all good.

What exactly does sacred mean?
Sacred means that the activity is
special and different enough from
your other activities that you
recognize it as so. Sacred means
that the activity is meaningful,
important to you, and connected to something greater than yourself,
but you cannot quite put it into words or explain it clearly to others,
unless they are a part of the sacred moment. It is a feeling or a

knowing. As my teenage son Golden said to me so poignantly, "It is what it is."

What are rituals? Rituals are meaningful activities you do with regularity in your home, religious community, work space, or society based on expectations, rules, or personal desires. They are meaningful on different levels depending upon who created them, how many people perform the rituals, and what role each person plays in the ritual. Rituals are different than chores or routines because they physically express our beliefs, values, feelings, or deeper concerns.

Let's put the two words together to have yet another tool to pull out of the wellness toolkit. When we light a candle while having our daily bath with the intention to pray and seek solace or meditation, it is a sacred ritual through everyday action. My auntie lights incense before going to bed, while saying her prayers, softly. My husband and I have a sacred daily task of whoever gets up last makes the bed so that even a glance of the peaceful, uncluttered bedroom from any other room in the house is enough of a respite from the rest of the chaotic day, a sanctuary in a glance. Smell the coffee deeply before taking the first sip. Sacred living through everyday actions need not be grand, but it will fill us with a needed wholeness that may be missing from our lives.

Before my kids went to sleep when they were little, I sang them two songs: the first song was one I made up years ago when I was a teenager at the school for the performing arts, a lullaby named *Sweet Dreams*. The second one was *Sunrise, Sunset* from *Fiddler on the Roof*. Those were our prayers and rituals before bedtime, sacred to our family dynamics. I worked at a hotel restaurant most evenings when they were younger (and I still do), so on my days off with them we always had a plan set in stone.

***

"It is only in stillness that one finds transformation."
—Lao Tzu

After the efforts and process, the stillness and rest provide a space for growth and deep understanding of what just occurred. Sometimes it takes years of effort before a breakthrough. Think of how many years it takes before one is finished with schooling. Then we physically, mentally, and spiritually make sense of it all. This happens after it is all over. Usually one takes a break, a rest, a season off, a vacation. Then the plan of what to do next reveals itself like a winter cloak being shed from one's shoulders for the first time in the spring.

Galina's Story

Galina was a gypsy of sorts. Her mom was a single mom and they moved from town to town in Indiana, picking up jobs waiting tables or cleaning homes for cash, under the table. Galina helped her mom from an early age, after school and on weekends. It was the only childhood she knew. She loved peering out the Greyhound bus windows as the terrain sped by them when they changed living arrangements. Galina had a sense of freedom from moving so much, and her mom was her anchor. The time spent together was a deep, loving, positive support system in the ever changing world.

One day while her mom was at the grocery store gathering cleaning supplies, a regular cleaning client came to the apartment. The man said that he wanted to pay Galina's mom for the week. Galina was fifteen years old, so she was old enough to be home alone. She let him in the apartment, and unfortunately he softly talked dirty, and began to touch Galina inappropriately. She pulled away abruptly, told him to stop, and yelled for him to get out of her home, now. He began to say softly and sweetly, "Come on, you know you like it..."

Luckily for Galina, her mom returned a few minutes later and freaked out on the guy, who fled the building in embarrassment. Soon after, the ladies were on the road again.

I first met Galina at the gym I went to, when she was in her late teens. She was a student in one of my spinning classes. We chatted often about fitness goals, and one day we decided to meet up for coffee at my home. One thing she kept mentioning over and over again was how impressed she was with my lack of clutter. I asked her why. She said that when the man violated her body boundaries as a kid, she began collecting things. Her way of coping with people and situations crossing boundaries was to create a huge physical barrier between her and men. Galina's mom continued to move them from town to town and it became harder and harder to move with so much stuff to pack and carry.

After Galina graduated high school, she went to a community college, and got her own place. She was working in a retail clothing store. Galina told me she now had too many clothes (employee discount). Galina asked me to help her de-clutter her apartment. Talk about a pack rat. Wow. When I saw her apartment, I could barely get through the hall to her living room. New clothes with tags on them were strewn everywhere, and boxes upon boxes lined every room.

As we worked through her fears and memories, we used the *Negative Thought Pot*. We also resolved the fact that those thoughts do not serve her anymore. She had to clear the clutter to make space for the right person to come into her life as a partner. It was easier for her to not have company (men) over or to have dates because she had the built-in excuse of her apartment being too messy.

Galina eventually gave loads of stuff away to charity, and had a garage sale where she met her fiancée!

When I come home from work at night I cannot go to bed when I see dishes in the sink or the Japanese screen around the desk in array. I wash the dishes, fix the screen in just the right position, wash the kitchen table, oil the wood with lemon essential oil, and kiss the children on their foreheads. I throw another load of dirty wash in the washing machine and then feel it is my sanctuary again. There is enough order to go to bed. I see myself as one of the little elves in the classic fairy tale, *The Elves and the Shoemaker*.

I think a cluttered home is a sign of a cluttered or unattended sanctuary. Your home is your sanctuary, and it is a reflection of what's going on inside of us. Sometimes it is a reaction to our past, and we want to fill up with so many things so we do not have to deal with the non-physical things. When we let go of clutter in our home, we create space. We allow the emptiness to be there. The empty space can be a bubble of peace, with room for more wonderful and new things to come into our lives, physically, mentally, emotionally, and spiritually. When we have space, we can attend to those things we need to see. We can finally *see*.

The perpetrators in these cases are also usually people who have been victims of physical, sexual, emotional, or verbal abuse in their own lives. It is a learned behavior. It is their go to power and control source. Typically sexual predators are not attracted to the people they are hurting. They desperately need therapy and healing as well. It doesn't minimize the tragedy, but it does help us understand where they started from.

An Invitation: write positive thoughts on a bathroom mirror

Using dry erase markers, write something positive and lovely about yourself on the bathroom mirror tonight to welcome your day tomorrow. You will be tired in the morning, so you may forget; sleepy and groggy, when you see yourself in the mirror, brushing your teeth, you won't be able to help but smile at your amazing start to the day. Change the words often and add more.

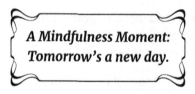

A Mindfulness Moment:
Tomorrow's a new day.

It's okay to lose your way sometimes, but you can also find your way back. You find your way back through connection, community, and ultimately, love.

Do you want to rest in peace before you rest in peace? If you were sexually molested in your life, letting go but not ever forgetting is a reality check. Then you can walk slowly and confidently towards your *Happy, Healthy You.*

Chapter Four

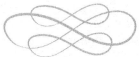

Facing Difficulties Head On ~ Confidence From Within

What if we could lose the old dogma of rehabilitation of the mind, body, and spirit, of fixing things *afterwards,* sometimes long afterwards? What if we face difficulties as they are happening to us, head on, and learn while we are coping *now*? This is a bold leadership move we see with our firefighters, police officers, the military, ER doctors, etc. Public service officers are seen as heroes, everyday heroes.

We regular folks can be everyday heroes too. We can be everyday, expected heroes to ourselves. It can come naturally, if we let our superior selves flow out naturally. In this chapter we will learn from people who made strong decisions and actions based upon the *now*, so that they had no regrets later. Sometimes they made good decisions that just came naturally to them, without really thinking about it based upon who they were, their personalities, their genetics...

"The time to repair the roof is when the sun is shining."
—John F. Kennedy

I love this quote. To me, this means we can make strong, bold moves when things are going well for us, but we have an inkling that there is a problematic situation coming our way. We can learn all we can from others' mistakes, choices, challenges, and how they recovered and rebounded in a successful manner (or not). This is an opportunity to *not* wait for the perfect moment to fix things. This is also the way of luck: preparation meeting opportunity.

Let's look at some inspiring stories of folks who faced their difficulties head on.

Chanel's Story: facing fears head on

Chanel hated her breasts from an early age. They were much too large for her small frame and height of five-feet-three inches. She developed early too: her period began at eight years old and her breast development was rapid. In high school, Chanel alternated binding her chest with ace bandages with wearing overlarge T-shirts on other days. She disappeared in her music, playing violin and singing the blues, old Dinah Washington songs from the 1930s.

She felt like she had been born in the wrong era. She often spoke to friends about being ready to die early, like she had a connection to the past that she could not remedy in this day and time, that she had to leave in order to do some of God's work in heaven. Chanel also spoke often of her past lives, especially in the medieval era. She definitely had the singing voice of an angel.

Chanel was also a serial bride. Men fell in love with her within weeks, asked her to marry them, and she would, usually within the first two months of dating. Once she told me, "If I'm good enough to sleep with, I'm good enough to marry." (We were friends since I was 15.)

Her underlying hatred of her breasts eventually manifested itself into breast cancer. She went through months of chemotherapy, a mastectomy, alternative eating methods, meditation, shamanic work, etc. After seven years of being cancer-free, the cancer returned with a vengeance. Now the cancer was in her brain, bones, and lymph glands. This time, however, the chemotherapy and experimental therapies did not help as much as the first time.

Chanel was completely calm and ready to be in spirit form, both times actually. It was the child she had borne that kept her from checking out of this world during her first bout with cancer. Chanel felt like she had so much more to offer the universe from the other side of life, the spiritual realm. Who could argue with that? Chanel was completely resigned and at peace with dying.

Chanel's daughter Raquel was eleven years old the second time her mother was diagnosed with widespread cancer. Raquel was at her mother's side during most of the treatments. They had plenty of time to bond, connect, reassure each other that love never dies, and to learn things from each other, even at the very end of the rope. Chanel used to say to me when we were teenagers, "The end of my rope is not the end of my hope."

Chanel passed away in Raquel's bedroom, in her daughter's arms. The dignity and grace with which Chanel lived her life, and then how she carried herself during the years of medical treatments, taught Raquel so much about this world. This was the gift and legacy that she left for her daughter. They kept grateful journals during those years, and the mother and daughter wrote little love notes back and forth. The box of notes was a constant reminder of a life well lived and well loved.

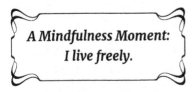

A Mindfulness Moment:
I live freely.

Raquel is now in her early twenties, strong, confident, and proud. She is sure of many things, mature beyond her years. Raquel is a real go-getter, and is successful in many areas of business. She is a real estate broker, the youngest ever to make the top sales tier for her company. Raquel is also fearless in trying new things, whether it is edgy hairstyles, extreme sports, or traveling alone to exotic places.

"With mom having to deal with the cancer and therapies for all those years, we learned to value what really mattered in this life. Mom taught me to face my own fears head on."

By regularly reviewing the notes and journals written during those difficult years, along with the calm preparedness for death and dying that Chanel possessed, she was able to give the gift of confidence and self-worth to her daughter at a young age.

Frannie's Story: the game of survival

Frannie is an immigrant from Vietnam, during the era of the Vietnam War. She was a child of eight years old when the sirens blared, and her parents gathered some food, clothes, and told their four kids that they had to go, *now*.

The family walked in the jungle for months on end, usually at night, in order to escape the watchful eyes of the soldiers and terrorists. While walking hundreds of miles, eating tree bark and insects for survival, Frannie turned the journey into a game with her brothers and sisters. They played games of who could be the quietest in the woods, which one of them could catch the most grasshoppers, and more games that they made up along the journey. Everything became a fun competition between the siblings. The games were also essential to their survival. It allowed the children to continue being children while developing great life skills.

The family walked all the way to Malaysia, eventually making their way to the United States, after living in a refugee camp for a few months. The bubbly personality, the friendly competitive spirit, and the appreciation for everything Frannie has now are direct results of those early difficult struggles. She chose, either consciously or subconsciously, to face the problems of food, survival, and family, head on. She now helps her coworkers see the positive side of everything in their daily lives, and helps them make light of minute hiccups during the work day. She recently won a company spirit award from the CEO of the bakery where she works. She was nominated by over half of the employees!

Frannie's uncanny sense of adventure and making light of a dark situation saved her life, and this personality trait has served her well during the years.

An Invitation: face your difficulties now, get happy now

This is a role-play exercise to do with a friend or family member.

Pretend that you are at the grocery store and the cashier is taking *waaaay* too long with the customer two people ahead of you. You are getting increasingly anxious and frustrated, because you have to pick up your son from school in thirty minutes. You thought you had timed everything perfectly, and now there's this huge wrench in your plans.

What can you do to solve this problem immediately and without being a total jerk to the rest of the people around you?

Act out three choices that yield the results you desire. Talk with the other person who is playing with you. Talk about why and how the choices you made are or are not effective.

Create your own second scenario with your partner. Act out the problems and solutions that will be effective immediately in the face of difficulty.

Now talk about a current real life situation that you want to conquer right now! Brainstorm ideas together with your partner.

After using the brainstorming tools out in the real world, call your role play partner and share how the real situation panned out.

Ursula's Story: no legs, full life

When I began practicing hot yoga about five years ago, a few people rode their bikes to the studio in Daly City, California. One petite, young woman with curly, black hair and muscles popping out everywhere almost knocked me over with her ninja skills on the bike as I walked half asleep toward the front door of the studio. "Oh, sorry!" she exclaimed. "Are you okay?" I told her I was fine, and I should have been more awake anyway. We chatted and introduced ourselves by name. Her name was Ursula.

As we went into the yoga room, I noticed she went to the front right corner, where the more advanced students liked to go. Then she did something I had never observed before. Ursula took off her legs. From the knees downwards, she unbuckled and unstrapped. The form and strength of her class was impeccable, untainted and unchanged by her prosthetic legs being on or off. I guess Ursula was a regular student because she was very muscular, her technique was amazing, and nothing held her back.

> **A Mindfulness Moment:
> Risk little, win little.**

In my mind, she was a wonder woman in the rest of her life as well, even though had I just met her. Ursula was a prime example of an everyday hero. Ursula had confidence from within. Whatever had brought her to the point in her life where I met her, she had to have met her difficulties head on or I would not have met her at all.

Mah's Story: I'm really ok with dying

When I sweat for ninety minutes in a hot yoga room with complete strangers, we build a community of trust. Trust that leaves the room with us.

My yoga friend Mah was waiting for a kidney transplant for quite some time and her dialysis was getting more frequent. Still, the strong and feisty woman was taking care of her meditation and self-care by coming to yoga almost daily. She was very powerful despite her kidney failure. I say this because this type of yoga is not an easy yoga. This yoga class was in a very hot, humid room, with muscle building poses that we would hold for a loooong time. (I invite you to join me any time, my treat. Then you will understand.)

Mah was wearing a dialysis belt and portal tube under her attractive yoga tank top which could only be seen once we were in the changing room. One day after class, in the shower area, I asked her about a transplant possibility and if I could volunteer to be tested for her.

Mah said, "Everybody in my immediate family has been tested and nobody is a match. Only close relatives can designate who gets a kidney if they want. You are not related to me. If you get tested and are a match for me, my number may not be up until two days from now. Someone whose number is up today and is a match with your kidney will get the call. Your kind gesture intended for me will go to someone else because you might be a match for them too."

That's how philanthropy with your organs works in the Northern California hospital systems. It is truly unconditional love. Mah didn't want me to have surgery, lose a kidney, and perhaps have medical issues later on in my life. She explained to me further, "I have lived a full life. My kids and grandkids have time ahead of them with lots to do and see. If they are a match and they give me their kidney, they will be laid up and weak for a long time. I don't want to hold them back. They have little kids and busy family schedules. I'm ready to go when the Lord wants me. I'm comfortable with that."

Her demeanor and resignation to be flowing with whatever healing or outcome the Universe provides to her is a big lesson for me.

The stories shared here are full of lessons for us all. Real hope, optimism, and choices are there for the taking. So, what are you going to do about your problem? Whether great or small, our problems still may keep us stuck in a certain state of mind. Thinking of answers is not enough. We must take action (without belittling any other party). Then we can move forward, focusing on our big, beautiful plans for our bright future.

This also refers back to contrasting drama to trauma, explained in detail in **Chapter 2**. Facing everyday drama head on seems relatively simple now, doesn't it? We can do this when we put things in their proper perspective, value the true strengths that have core meaning in our lives, and allow the fringe to remain on the fringe.

"I, not events, have the power to make me happy or unhappy today. I can choose which it shall be. Yesterday is dead, tomorrow hasn't arrived yet. I have just one day, today, and I'm going to be happy in it."
—Groucho Marx

An Invitation: a grounding object

Some of my most positive friends carry a grounding object with them all the time. When they feel anxiety or old feelings pop up that do not serve them, or remind them of a negative past, they hold onto that object. Try this technique yourself. Choose a beautiful stone, crystal or something small. Hold it for a few minutes to honor its purpose and set it up as your grounding tool. It may keep you calm, keep you grounded, and keep you remembering a special memory that was joyful and blissful. Perhaps a memory of laughter and good times with family will arise. Close your eyes for a few seconds and imagine something positive that allows you to let go of anxiety, fear, or bad memories, and replaces it with something wonderful.

Then perhaps the bad feelings, the anxiety, and the stress may dissipate quickly and easily because you have that grounding stone or crystal that you keep with you regularly. It is a new habit, a habit of courage, a habit that will serve your higher purpose and the new you, a *Happy, Healthy You.*

Just for a moment every day, instead of being pissed off that you were not born with the happy and giddy gene, pretend you were. Fake it. Put on the glitter, do 20 jumping jacks to get your blood pumping, say, "I love you," to yourself in the mirror with a ridiculous grin. Eventually the neural pathways in your brain will follow the repetitive actions and statements you are creating and you will begin to have new science literally follow the new belief systems. Well done. Welcome to a *Happy, Healthy You.*

Chapter Five

Unlucky in Love...Over and Over ~ Finally Free

"That's just how people – men, treat me."

Why do I hear this phrase over and over again from all of my single or suddenly single friends and family? To be completely honest with you, dear readers, it makes me feel a little bad to have such a long term, solid, strong relationship with my husband.

Wait a minute! Why should I feel bad about a good thing? I have been with my sweetheart for more than 25 years, and even though we have had ups and downs, like any long term relationship, we are committed, not giving in, and not giving up.

Relationships with our significant others give us the most rushes of joy and pain, that is, until we have children...then the children take over in the creation of giant swings of emotion in mama and papa. We are not chained to the same story over and over again. Let us hear about Rena's life.

Rena's Story

Rena was absolutely stunning. She was petite, with a size 24 inch waist and a size 34D bra. She was bubbly, energetic, *and* brilliant. In her high school and college classes she was a straight A student, but all of the attention from males was aimed at her chest, not stimulated by her intelligence. At 20 years old, she fell in love, became pregnant with twins, and gave up her schooling to raise a family. She got married at five months pregnant. Rena married five times and divorced five times. She eventually had five children, and she loved them fiercely.

When I met her, she told me nonchalantly that she was resigned to having bad relationships. She was at the point in her life where she expected people to treat her as less than a goddess, less than brilliant. I asked her, point blank, "Is it because you let them treat you badly, or because you choose men with whom you have an instinct that they will treat you badly? Do you have a natural flair or a preference for barbaric, macho men?" Perhaps she had bad luck...

This had been her repetitive relationship life. It turns out that she had been a child pageant star in her small home town in Tennessee. Boys and men focused on her as entertainment, the girl on their arms. She attracted those types of men toward her because that was all she knew.

It really does not matter when those experiences changed to being accustomed to poor behavior being directed towards her, but the fact is that it was happening over and over again.

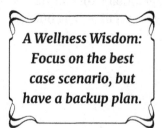

A Wellness Wisdom: Focus on the best case scenario, but have a backup plan.

The use of both negative and affirmative letters is a powerful tool in releasing the past emotions one feels are holding oneself back from one's future. I asked Rena to write a letter to her numerous boyfriends and past husbands as if they were one person. I told her to write to them including every little thing that was not okay with her and why. Then I asked her to write another letter to herself describing every quality she admired about herself, with or without a life partner, and if she had a life partner what those qualities in a partner looked like *now*.

The first letter Rena wrote she was instructed to mail to me at my address. She put it in the mailbox with a witness. The second letter, she was to address to herself, and once again, have a witness watch her put it into the mailbox, signed, sealed, and stamped.

When she received the letter to herself, she was to meet with me and open it in my presence. I told her to read it out loud to me. I repeated everything she wrote, sentence by sentence. Hearing someone else say the words aloud affirmed what her desires in a partner were. She was very clear and poignant in her writing.

I told her to save her affirmative letter in a drawer under her clothes, in a place where she could see the envelope peeking out every day when she got dressed. It was a great reminder of what goodness she embodied and what goodness she deserved. This is another tool from the wellness toolkit, like the *Negative Thought Pot*.

"You don't know a woman until you have had a letter from her."
—Ada Leverson, writer

I told her to devote *herself* to *herself*. When she did that, she finally felt like she could see the possibility of becoming whole again, complete, without another person to complete her. In many cases, that's when the universe sees us happy and how much energy and love we have to bring to the table. That is when the universe brings someone into our lives who is also happy and ready for a deep fulfilling relationship. That is the Universe confirming a *Happy, Healthy You*.

The other letter speaking to the bad relationship situations, she was to tear up and flush down the toilet right in front of me. Neither she nor I needed to hear her *lack* anymore, perhaps because she lived through it!

An Invitation: letters to Santa Claus & to yourself

Write a letter to your wrongdoers documenting every bad thing that has happened to you that you feel has shaped your poor choices. Tell the person or persons what was not loving, what was painful, and why. Tell them the behavior *was* and *is not* acceptable. Address the envelope to Santa Claus, #1 North Pole Lane, North Pole. Do not put your return address on the envelope. Put it in the mailbox. The physical act of sending it off into the world wide postal system is a real act of change.

Do you really care who opens and reads it after you put it in the mailbox? If you are comfortable and strong enough to address the letter to the person or persons who have treated you less-than... you are free to do that. Just know that they may want to reach out to you to make amends, and you have to be prepared mentally and emotionally to deal with that aspect of forgiveness.

Write a second letter. Define exactly what you want in a partner or for your life. Mail it to yourself. It is liberating and validating to have a final closure and actually a new beginning in this way. This is an actionable step in dealing with the problem of being treated with less than the highest honor, respect, and love.

Rena had to work on her self esteem in order to realize what was acceptable and not acceptable in her current life. Regardless of how men have treated her in the past, Rena is valuable and important to the world. When she has moments of doubt about her value as a woman, I suggested that she focus on being a good example of a strong and deserving goddess for her children's sake. They will mirror the confident behavior she exhibits, resulting in well developed, happy, and self-assured adults.

That being said, sometimes we just have to fake it 'til we make it. Even if Rena still has elements of self-doubt, by outwardly expressing confidence, over and over again, I do believe it will rub off on her. I believe that Rena will care about herself more as time goes on, and she will intrinsically *know* she matters a whole lot to the people around her. Eventually Rena will believe that she is worthwhile and capable of growth, and that she has a joyful, healthy future in front of her.

Years ago, I remember preparing a private room in a restaurant for a small university alumni dinner party. I was rubbing furiously on my shirt pocket with club soda and a sponge, trying to get an ink stain out. I walked into the managers' office, pointed to my shirt, and lifted my hands up in frustration. Arnold smiled at me, and said calmly, "It doesn't have to be so hard, KJ. You still have time. Go to the uniform room and see if they are still open. There's still time to change." Wow. Arnold gave me great advice, and such a simple solution too. Life can be like that too. There is still time to change, if you want to, and if you *go downstairs and do the changing.*

"It's never too late in — fiction or in life — to revise."
—Nancy Thatcher, writer

A Constant State of Fear

Sometimes we don't even realize this, but we may live in a constant state of fear due to different levels of abandonment in our early years. People we love move away, our parents or relatives break up, the sibling who is older moves out for college, a loved one dies. The feeling of abandonment may make it harder for us to find *the one* later on in our lives. This feeling may manifest itself in our lives by us choosing not to date at all, or going from one relationship to another in rapid succession, leaving them (so they don't leave us first), or choosing people who treat us as less than our full gloriousness!

Our minds and hearts do have a great potential for healing. I believe that if we give ourselves half a chance, we can recover with resilience from fear-based living in stagnation.

Yvonne's Story

Yvonne had witnessed brutal death a couple of times during her childhood. She was the youngest of four children, living in the inner city of Chicago. Her mother and father were in a committed relationship, but not married. At age five, she watched her father die in her mother's arms, after a drive-by shooting outside her apartment building. Then when she was eleven years old, her mother died suddenly of previously undiagnosed cancer.

Yvonne had deep seated feelings of abandonment. Within weeks of her mother's passing, bad things seemed to happen to her over and over. Her school burned down. Her dog got run over. Her keyboard broke. Her favorite doll that her mother had given her lost an arm. Eventually she became used to the darkness. She thought that this was her lot in life. She identified herself as the bad talisman, that she, herself, was bad luck to those around her. In her eleven year old mind, if she was *bad luck*, then she must be *bad*. For this young survivor, death made her experience guilt (unfounded of course).

I met Yvonne in a vitamin shop when she was in her twenties. "I'm tainted," she told me one day. "Everything and everyone that gets close to me has bad luck. I feel like there is a dark cloud hanging over my soul. I don't know why."

About six months after Yvonne's mother passed away, she and her siblings were unfortunately split up. She thought this was her fault too. She went to live with her maternal grandmother in another state. She was devastated to have to start over again, and leave the few people who were close to her. Her grandmother loved Yvonne dearly, but resented having to raise another child at this point in her life.

Unfortunately, for Yvonne, no grief counseling or therapy was offered after her mother's death, as all the energy was focused on the day-to-day tasks of caring for the four children, and then the attention was on the big move. Over time, she became increasingly quiet and introverted to the point where she rarely spoke.

Her elderly grandmother thought this was a rite of passage, part of being a moody teenager. What her octogenarian grandmother didn't realize was that this was a case of classic dissociation, zoning out into another world, withdrawing from society and those close to her. Yvonne was not given the opportunity to release her grief, her guilty feelings, her abandonment issues, or her thinking that somehow she had provoked bad luck in the very air around her.

"I think the one lesson I have learned is that there is no substitute for paying attention."
—Diane Sawyer, journalist

I asked Yvonne to write down what made her happy on a daily basis, or from a memory in her past. The happy activities or moments could be big or small, mundane or monumental. She was to write down three things a day for a week.

When she saw the long list of things that made her happy, she could no longer deny her present opportunity to be happy. Yvonne saw at last that she deserved to be with another good human being for a long time, despite the $#!+ that had happened in the past. The fear of someone leaving, or of her leaving became easier to give up as a normal, expected behavior. As time went on, Yvonne began to see things from a different perspective. Different expectations began to emerge. As the saying goes, "Every dark cloud has a silver lining." (I add that there is usually rain before a rainbow.)

When Yvonne saw in her own handwriting that insignificant things could bring her moments of joy, she woke up to the possibilities that she, herself, could bring others to experience joy, and that she was not a bad luck omen after all. After three months of writing joy lists, Yvonne felt like the dark cloud had lifted from her shoulders.

In her late twenties, Yvonne found true love in a long term relationship. Her fear of abandonment and intimacy faded. She is now able to be warm and close to those she formerly was distant towards. Things are looking up.

"Your mind works for you. You don't work for your mind. If you don't mind, it doesn't matter."
—Michael, yoga instructor

An Invitation: daily joy

For seven consecutive days, write down three things that give you joy. Do this right before retiring for the night, so the last things you remember before sleeping are happy thoughts. Set the list next to the bed on your side table. When you feel down on yourself or disconnected from the good things going on in your life, reach for the list and read it silently or out loud. You have so much untapped joy. This is just the tip of the iceberg. Go deep. (Notice that this is not a grateful journal. That is another exercise that we will use later on in this book.)

Some of us need a buddy or two to help us meet our goals in life. Challenge someone else to do this joyful exercise with you. This is a great way to build trust around abandonment issues and to build a support system at the same time. If you have someone to whom you are accountable, and they to you, it works even better. Over time, you will become more accountable to yourself.

Somehow, and in some way, we *can* make pretty out of an ugly situation. I encourage you to allow the letters to yourself and the notebook of happy, joyous moments to act as a personal bridge out of negativity into positivity.

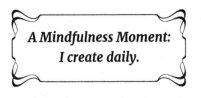

A Mindfulness Moment:
I create daily.

Our brains and hearts are connected, no matter what we go through in our lives. I believe we chose to be here on this earth and at this particular time. I believe we made an agreement with the Universe, God, the One That Is, Love Itself, to have these challenges on earth, so that we may grow. Good or bad, it is all growth and understanding. The heart will help us understand what the brain analyzes. Then, the heart sets us afire under the feelings. I don't want us to deny the feelings underneath the facts. I want us to bloom from them, to take action, to do something. We can do more than just acknowledge that *this* or *that* happened.

Blossom and bloom into a *Happy, Healthy You.*

Chapter Six

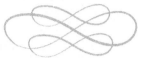

Work Place Challenges ~ We All Have Them...

Read the following questions and see if they are true or false for you:

- Are you not being taken seriously at work when brainstorming ideas in a group?

- Do you raise your hand at department meetings and then get overlooked?

- Are your contributions not being implemented and you are not given an explanation why?

- Are your contributions *being* implemented, but you are not given credit?

- Are you constantly in conflict with the same coworker or coworkers?

- Does someone just irk you, get on your nerves, get under your skin, just by *being*, and you can't tell him or her off because you are at work?

We all want to feel like we have value and have a great deal to offer our place of employment, whether our job is restocking the shelves at the corner store or piloting a revolutionary software program that will change the way we prepare our IRS tax returns forever. Whether in a large collaborative work space or a small mom and pop operation, we want to feel like *what we do matters* (See **Chapter 8**.). What we say and how we say it really does matter. It can mean the difference between keeping our job and losing it. There is a fine dance between authentic expression in the workplace and going overboard. There is also a fine line between holding one's tongue and withholding communication altogether, commonly called repression.

At work, we have to maintain a professional demeanor when expressing our feelings in the heat of the moment. To be effective, we cannot just fly off the handle like we do sometimes at home (unfortunately) with our kids or our significant other. It is considered unprofessional. I encourage my clients to breathe deeply ten times through the nasal passages to slow their emotions down before expressing themselves during conflict. If this does not work for them, I advise them to take a bathroom break. Sometimes a change of physical location will give one a different point of view, a few minutes to cool down, and a chance to meditate on a solution rather than focus on the problem or the personal conflict.

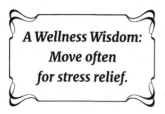

A Wellness Wisdom:
Move often
for stress relief.

On the other hand, when we completely hold in our reactions to problems, and do not express ourselves at all at work, it is counterproductive. Repressed feelings in the workplace can be handled by going for a run, a kickboxing class, yoga, a hike in the woods, a walk at the beach, weightlifting, or any activity that gets the heart pumping. The energy that was pent up can be released naturally and powerfully, used for a good purpose, and the activity is healthy for our own physical and mental strength. Then the solution to the work place challenge may come in a natural flow and the person may be ready to share his or her feelings without freaking out.

Repressed feelings in the work place environment over the long term may turn someone into an introvert, or into an antisocial person. The individual may turn to food for comfort, or to alcohol, drugs, or to unsafe sex; they may become sad, or suffer from anxiety, and this may eventually lead to the blues or depression. He or she may not perform their best at work and may not be able to focus. This is a restricting way to live one's life. It affects the whole life, in and out of the work environment. It does not feel good and will not lead to success or happiness inside or outside of the work-place. We need a plan of action.

I suggest if you feel you cannot fully express who you are at work in a conflict or in a meeting, or if you don't feel comfortable dealing with conflict at work, seek out others who seem to have it all together in that area. Ask for advice from someone you admire. Go to the Human Resources department and ask for help.

The best way to express yourself in a timely and level-headed manner is to write down on a note pad the conflict that irks you and what ideas or solution you have to offer. That way you will be seen as a helper rather than as a complainer. That is positive energy. Positive energy is exponential and contagious. Bring the solution to your supervisor as soon as you can. Don't wait too long to seek out assistance, or it may seem like everybody forgot about the problem but you.

Particularly closed off individuals are those who I would call shy. Perhaps he or she was raised as an only child. Perhaps he or she was naturally drawn to reading in the bedroom, curled up with a good book instead of playing at the park with all of the other neighborhood kids. We need to show compassion and empathy in the work place to those folks, because we do not yet know the whole story, not until he or she decides to share.

As a child grows into an adult, the responsibilities increase exponentially. Most of us hope to go to college or trade school, find a passion, a career, and go for it! Along the way, we come across folks in our schooling or work who don't jibe with our groove. We are too different. Our cultures, our upbringings, our attitudes, our personalities, whatever...seems to bring division and conflict and tension rather than unity in the interactions, over and over again.

When we are at work (or school) and we have conflicts or tensions with other coworkers, it may not always be blatantly obvious. Sometimes those feelings may be simmering just under the surface.

To society at large, the challenges may not seem like such a big deal. After all, we aren't married to our colleagues. Usually they aren't part of our immediate family or part of our inner circle of influence. The amount of hours spent together daily, however, can and does influence our lives as a whole. Sometimes our coworkers become closer to us than blood relatives. Work place relationships are pretty intense at times. Tempers may flare, and the pain is very real when conflict occurs. This is part of life's journey too. We may have anger and frustration and ask ourselves again and again, "Why me?" As much as we want to be logical, it is an emotional experience. At times, there may be the feeling like there is no path through the murky swamp to the grassy knoll on the other side.

Ronald's Story: I don't care if I get fired

One day, I was on the bus, and I overheard a conversation between two friends. Let's call them Ronald and James. Ronald exclaimed, "Ooooh, I think I am going to explode! Why does my colleague always _____, when he/she knows that I don't like that, and I don't expect to be treated in that way? Sometimes, I swear that he/she does this $#!+ on purpose. The next time it happens, I'm going to the big boss, or to Human Resources, or I will take it into my own hands. I don't even care if I get *fired.*"

Does this sound familiar to you? The response from James was, "Just let it go, man. It is just not worth the stress and energy you are putting forward. Put it in God's hands and walk away from that mess."

Great advice from a good friend, for sure, but I didn't get to hear the rest of the conversation. As I stepped down from the bus, I was thinking, "Yes, yes, but *how*? How is one supposed to let that constant $#!+ go?"

I thought deeply about my own work status, how I pretty much have made a family out of my coworkers. After all, we spend most evenings in that one space together. I get along with almost all of them. When someone does something to get under my skin, over and over, it seems intentional, absolutely. But perhaps, just perhaps, they do not even realize what they are doing!

I say the first step is to have a calm conversation with the individual. If this still does not get through to the other person, then give it some time, like a couple of weeks. If you still feel annoyed because the behavior does not stop, then I advise you to speak with a supervisor. Allow the manager to take the burden off of your shoulders. If there is a sort of retaliation towards you, then consider having a conversation with Human Resources. In my experience, once the Human Resource department hears the word harassment, they will step in and have a resolution for you pretty darn quickly.

My last resort, and I have done this in my work place, is to literally tell myself the other person does not exist. If they no longer exist, they hold no emotional power over me.

We give so much credence to our work lives because we have a strong self-identity within that space. When we meet strangers at a party, eventually the conversation veers towards finding out what the other person does for a living. The question itself, "What do you do for a living?" implies that what we do in order to make money is who we are and how we live our life. The very term *living* means that it is how we identify ourselves. It is a cultural belief that we *are* what we do for a living.

When seeking a mate, we ask them what their job is, and evaluate them in a way that shows us whether they can support us in a financial way, or if they can intellectually support our own career ambitions.

When I was a little kid, one of the first questions grownups asked me upon meeting me was, "What do you want to be when you grow up?"

Be? I will still *be* me. I want to continue *being me.* Really, what they were asking was what career path or job did I want to pursue? I find myself doing the same thing to my children's friends. It is part of our belief system in this society that our jobs, our careers, and our work are so, so important to our self worth. It makes sense then, that we have a high value judgment and energy investment in our career or job, as well as judging others based upon their work life.

Likewise, when we lose our jobs, we feel like someone has punched us in the stomach, like our sails have no wind. Well, who am I now? I have been fired, laid off, cut back, cut down, left behind....I am lost. Maybe I *am* replaceable. I am not as valuable as I thought. I am *a nobody.* The wheels in our mind begin spinning, and we may spiral downward if we do not have a strong sense of self worth, if we do not have a support system outside of work that is unconditionally loving.

We must realize that work is but a facet of our lives, and not our entire existence.

My Story: I cannot get in others' heads

Servers at my workplace tip out the bartenders and bussers at the end of their shift, after cashing out the nightly report.

There is one bartender at the hotel where I work who used to be friendly with me. Let's call him Brandon. After almost twenty years of working in the same department, you might think we were like family at best, and like friends, or friendly and professional at the very least. Unfortunately this bartender had financial problems outside of work. When the tech industry was booming on the stock exchange, he purchased an apartment in another country on a credit card, and then the stock market took a dive. Our restaurant and bar was not busy for a long time.

Brandon began to get moody, and began taking tables outside of his designated bartender territory. He also transferred checks to his number, which basically was stealing. One other bartender took him to Human Resources multiple times to try to get these actions to stop.

One evening, I was released early because business was slow. I told the manager I would cash out after changing out of my uniform and come back upstairs to tip out the staff. A few minutes later Brandon nearly knocked me over in the *ladies' locker room*, insisting I had not tipped him out yet! I was in my middle of changing and this was totally inappropriate. I stated, "Would you mind if I finished changing clothes first? I am still on the clock and haven't received my tips yet." Brandon should have known this because bartenders are the ones who give the servers their nightly tips from their cashier drawers.

Of course, I had to report the inappropriate behavior as harassment to Human Resources. I have calmly and continuously treated Brandon with professional respect, saying, "Thank you," after every drink, every time. This is common bar culture. He even went to complain to the managers over the years that saying "thank you" was rude because he wanted me to not talk to him at all. Of course, they dismissed him as being unreasonable and as being a bit stressed over his unfavorable life choices.

I had to back away and look at the bigger picture, even though inside I wanted to kick Brandon in the balls! We do not know what things are going on inside other folks' minds, hearts, and souls. What if he was an artist who dreamed of retiring in a little village in Europe, painting away his senior years in that apartment? Imagine the internal turmoil and disappointment. What if he had to take care of ailing parents and saw the far off apartment as a refuge, a sanctuary? Now, his dreams would be dashed, and he would have to work on his future all over again.

I went to Human Resources and took care of the legality of the offense, taking care of *me*, without letting the whole thing turn into a cycle of hate and *tit for tat*. I now treat Brandon as I always did, with grace and professionalism. I do not let the games he continues to play get under my skin, but to be honest, if I run into this person when we are both retired, I may speak my mind (and I hope he wears a protective cup).

An Invitation: breathe in power, let go of reaction

Practice this meditation for 60 seconds before hitting the work place. Sit in the bathroom stall, car, locker room, etc. Count upwards and backwards to ten three times, with inhalation and exhalation through the nose. This calms the nervous and circulatory systems, as well as the respiratory system, and lowers blood pressure. Say to yourself at the end, three times, "_____ is not a factor in my life. _____ holds no power over me, physically, emotionally, or spiritually. I welcome a joyful work day."

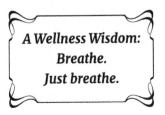

A Wellness Wisdom:
Breathe.
Just breathe.

I have found that this exercise, when practiced with regularity, resulted in the person no longer talking to me at all. We were like two cars on the same freeway, in different lanes with the windows rolled up. To me, that individual disappeared. What a relief.

Some of you are thinking, "I can't do that. We have to collaborate on projects. We have to communicate in order to get the actual work done." Focus on the work then, not the person. It is as if the words are coming from the heavens or another dimension, rather than from the coworker who is driving you mad. If you are willing to pretend and suspend reality, you will see that working together will be doable. Trust me. I have done exactly that.

"The trouble with being in the rat race is that even if you win, you're still a rat."
—Lily Tomlin, actor, comedian

I do not entirely agree with the above statement. When in business, any business, whether you are the owner, management, or the hourly laborer, you can work with compassion and still make a profit. I call this **compassionate capitalism**. There is a way to be a money maker in our world and still take care of people's hearts. (There is a way to eat abundantly and enjoy treats without sabotaging your own greater good. See Chapter 1.)

Taking Away the Competitive Edge When It is Not Necessary

People at work come to me often to help them with their own issues, whether they are work related or not. I taught wellness workshops at my work place for a few consecutive months a while back. Many folks outside of my department see me as a friend and confidante. During my workshops, I always speak of my personal struggles with aging, obesity, parenting, etc. I find that when I am open enough with others to be honest about my own challenges, it sets the tone for them to have real and effective communication with me about their own life challenges.

Showing vulnerability allows team members to realize that they are not isolated. It shows that we each have been given special strengths to deal with our unique problems. The universal themes that surround us while working through stuff at work (or anywhere, really) are proof that we *can* make it through to the other side of the darkness, and that we *can* rely on others for care and support (on many levels).

Being open to change is not a sign of weakness. I think it is a sign of honor, a willingness to muster up the courage to do whatever it takes to have the results one wants. This works on the job, and in life.

Being mindful that change is inevitable in the work place also allows us to be receptive to the input of others. We can set aside our competitive edge for something greater. When we are used to being rebellious, and have a history of bucking authority, we feel that it makes us appear tough and resilient. Just for a moment, imagine that you are on the receiving end of the toughness. That tough attitude may make you appear like a jerk to others. There is a difference between behaving like a leader, one who is independent, creative, and powerful, and just appearing like an inflexible bully. How do you want to be remembered when you retire?

"To be meek, patient, tactful, modest, honorable, brave, is not to be either manly or womanly; it is to be humane."
—Jane Harrison, scholar

Things will always irk us in life. We feel disrespected at times. We must think about the reasons and steps that brought us to this particular environment in the first place. Are those reasons enough now to stay where we are? What if we are bitter? What if we actually despise going to work each day? Can we change our attitude and the work aura with the _Negative Thought Pot_? Do we have enough money saved up to follow our next passion and path? Slowing down long enough to consider all of the options is important. I am a list maker. I list the pros and cons when making career changes. Then I pray on it before sleeping at night. Usually after a few days of this the correct path reveals itself to me.

Work place challenges do get fixed when the individuals have internal self respect. It has to start there. I must respect and love myself to a point where I am stable and confident (not cocky) in who I am as a human being first, then confident in what I have to offer a coworker, company, or anybody, really. What do I want to be when I grow up? I want to be a _Happy, Healthy Me_.

Chapter Seven

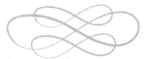

Humor as a Healer ~ Bring Your "A" Game to the Tickle Challenge

When we are in the middle of an emotional storm caused by trauma or drama, most of us cannot see through the mess. In the middle of a hurricane, however, there is the eye; there is the eerily calm and silent space at the center. There may be $#!+ happening all around you, or to you, but we do have the internal fortitude to breathe deeply and calmly and get through it.

My favorite aunt, Aunt Lulu, who passed away years ago, used to start out by being very quiet when she was worried, stressed, or ill. When the $#!+ hit the fan, she would get quiet, then after a while she would begin giggling. Then the giggles would grow into full-blown laughter, lasting ten minutes or more.

Usually when traumatic things occurred in her large family, we would rally around her. All of her favorite nieces and nephews came to be with her family when her house burned down. Her laughter was contagious. Before you knew it, all twenty of us were rolling on the ground with deep belly laughter, tears streaming down our faces.

Organically and naturally, a logical and methodical solution presented itself after the laughter session. The house burning down was not *her* burning down, and she and her family were miraculously fine.

Aunt Lulu didn't know about the theory of humor therapy as a coping and healing tool, but this was what she did to cope. She blessed the mess with laughter. Humor was her ally, and it carried her far and wide through her tough times. Humor allows us to laugh at ourselves and the situation, at each other, and at life in general. It helps us remove judgment and negativity.

When I was a teenager, my friends and I would walk to the park after school and play Frisbee. When we rested on the grass, we would lie in a big, sloppy pile or circle. We would put our heads on one another's tummies. One person would begin an intentional laugh, therefore making the other person's head bob up and down. Then the head bobbing person would begin laughing for real, and it continued until everybody was laughing hysterically. All felt right with the world after those afternoons.

Have you ever been told as a young child to be very quiet? Then you and your friends somehow caught the giggles? It was a natural coping technique for the body to deal with the pressure of being told, as a little kid, to be so quiet and serious. After all, that is not very natural to the body when young.

Laughter Yoga: it is a real therapy

Laughter therapy has been used in many cases of mental and physical suffering. Laughter therapy is also called laughter yoga. It was developed in India in 1995 by Dr. Madan Kataria. It involves playful exercises and breathing exercises meant to trigger laughter. There are laughter yoga centers all over the world hosting classes based upon his healing techniques.[8]

Laughter assists in relieving chronic pain by releasing endorphins and other feel good hormones. These are natural painkillers. Laughter yoga is also useful in stress management. Since laughter is naturally contagious, it benefits not only the sufferer, but those surrounding the person in need as well. Laughter oxygenates your body and brain. Deep belly laughs make us breathe deeper.

Clinical research in Bangalore, India and in the United States has shown that the body cannot distinguish between real laughter and fake laughter.[9] We receive the physiological benefits either way. When we release the feel-good hormones after laughing, levels of the stress hormones cortisol and epinephrine are reduced. Reduction in these hormone levels are a good thing (unless you are being chased by a tiger).

Smiling has also been shown to be useful in happy hormone release, whether it is a real smile or a fake smile. It strengthens the immune system and widens the passageways from the nose and throat, which is beneficial if one has a cold or allergies.

> ***"Smile high! Smile low! Smile everywhere you go!"***
> —Dr. Seuss

I work with a charming Spaniard named Jose. When I first met him years ago, he walked and talked quickly, with lots of natural energy and vibrancy. His smile was brilliant and honest. I told him, "I love your smile." He replied, "It's yours."

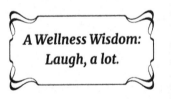

A Wellness Wisdom:
Laugh, a lot.

I never forgot his words. I think about those words when I am having a blah day, or just going through the motions of my errands and responsibilities. The power of those words, the gift of his smile to me, meant everything to me in that moment. Jose may not read this book, or even know his impact upon my life, but that's what we humans can be and are to each other: everything. Imagine what your smile or gentle gesture may mean to another person, especially if they are feeling fragile or vulnerable. I think we all do kindnesses that we do not even realize the impact of, and that gives me hope even during the dark times.

When I think of my own life and deep belly laughter moments, it has always been in conjunction with other people. I have maintained mostly good feelings toward others, and ultimately I feel connected to them when we can laugh together.

Bob's Story: tsunami jokes

Bob was working as a cook in Thailand, at a beach resort. The open kitchen was next to the water, literally on the beachfront. When the tsunami was coming in, nobody noticed until it was too late. The waves crashed upon the shores and the kitchen was suddenly a crashing mess of pots, pans, knives, glassware, and food.

As fast as he could, Bob shouted to his colleagues to swim away from the water, to swim upwards toward the highlands. This was the direction of the waves too. He began singing folk songs and telling knock-knock jokes from his childhood. It kept his breathing regular, and he didn't panic.

Those around him caught his voice in the air and joined him. They sang and laughed while they swam to higher ground and safety. Laughter was their immediate savior, their coping tool. The bonds created by humor and music literally saved their lives.

The people Bob worked with and survived with rebuilt their homes near each other after the tsunami. They became close as family. The humor and mutual respect between them can be felt just by being in their presence.

An Invitation: make yourself laugh

Think about a decision you have to make. It can be great or small. Now change the situation so the people involved are cartoon characters. Think about how they would interact in a Saturday morning cartoon. See the humor through the seriousness. Now, do this for another decision that you must make. It may be as simple as going to the grocery store and choosing what your family will have for dinner, or as complicated as where you will move and live in the next year.

Go onto the internet and look up America's Funniest Home Videos. Just a few old episodes will have you rolling with laughter. Better yet, watch the clips with a friend or family member. You will experience the humor even more deeply. Just as *misery loves company*, so does humor. The world will seem like a sunnier, funnier place.

An Invitation: tickle time

Do you have kids? Do you have friends or family members who have kids? I'm talking about little kids here, about ages 3-10. Borrow some *right now*. Have you ever played tickle monster? Have you ever tested your laugh limits? Tickle monster is where you get your hands up and mimic tickling the person opposite you, moving closer and closer until you are actually tickling them. You take turns, until all mayhem breaks loose and everybody is tickling everybody else. The anticipation time when you see the tickler coming toward you creates a giggle or laugh, even before anyone is touched.

Testing your laugh limits is where one person lies face down on the floor and the people around him or her, ever so lightly brush their fingertips all over the person's back, arms, or legs. The ticklers quietly count the seconds to see how long it takes before the victim laughs. The winner is the person who has the longest control time. First, we control ourselves before we allow ourselves to lose control in this safe and healing way to laughter.

Tickle time is so effective in showing us the joy kids and laughter bring to the world. I find that it teaches us the life lesson of how to let loose from our adult problems some of the time. We really need this.

I crack myself up every day! My internal dialogue leaves me chuckling, especially during my hot yoga class. I think to myself, during the poses, "You want me to put *what, where?* And hold that for sixty seconds? *That's* hilarious."

I liken the internal humor in my hot yoga class to being pregnant. It is tough going sometimes during the journey, yet at the end, you are glad you did it. They both involve copious amounts of patience, self-discipline, and a healthy outlook, as well as fluids, smells, and noises coming out of every part of my body.

Another humorous mind game that occurs within me during hot yoga is renaming the guided poses as the teacher calls the directions out. When I hear, "Nose to toes," I substitute it with, "Hocus, pocus," or, Focus, focus." When the teacher says, "Turn around and lie down," my mind changes it to, "Kick your boyfriend out of town." When the teacher instructs, "Breathe, just breathe," I switch the phrase to, "Leave, just leave." Perhaps after a few years of hot yoga classes, I have learned to inject internal humor into the difficult practice. Otherwise, I might just cry.

I remember when I was a kid the funniest movies my father would take us to were not comedies. They were R rated movies my mother did not want him to see because they were inappropriate and she was more conservative than he was. So he would load us up in the car and drive five minutes away instead of walking down the street. That way my mom thought we were going to a far away movie theater. We would enjoy our popcorn and soda, pretending to watch the film, but slyly watch our father watching the film. He was enjoying Bo Derek in *Tarzan and in 10, Porky's,* and other inappropriate films for a girl of elementary school age. I was laughing so hard one time with my siblings that pop (soda) came dripping out from my nostrils. My father loved being naughty in a kids' manner with us, loved laughing, making jokes, and making us laugh. Perhaps that's one reason he lived until age 93.

"You grow up the day you have your first real laugh at yourself."
—Ethel Barrymore, actor

Humans have used laughter as a coping and healing technique for a long, long time. It has been used in shamanic healing ceremonies all around the world for millennia. Humor gives us hope, an optimistic view of life and its challenges, as well as a connectedness to others. Lighten up for a *Happy, Healthy You.*

Chapter Eight

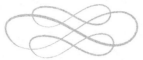

Surviving or Thriving After the Loss of a Loved One? Good Grief

In earlier chapters, we saw examples of coping and then recovering after the death of a loved one. In this chapter we will look into this more deeply. Coping with any problem is how one deals with and processes the situation immediately. Recovering or healing from a problem is more long term, and requires more thought and more work. After all, almost everybody experiences the death of a loved one during their life, usually multiple times. Most of us experience the deaths of the elders in our family before we die ourselves.

Those of us who are watching over the dying usually try to move bravely throughout the process. We do not want the dying loved one to sense our own fears, anger, loss of control, or our impending grief. We also do not want the other people around us to sense that we are "losing it."

We try to merge the spiritual and practical aspects of death with a sense of grace and dignity. Who arranges the funeral or memorial? Who inherits the stuff and who inherits the debt? Who does all the cleaning up and clearing out of the home? There are so many things to do and so little time to do it all, but most of all, we want to sit by the bedside and caress the hand or cheek of our beloved and say over and over, "I love you forever." We want to reminisce, to keep it light when we can. Some of us put up a courageous front and some of us completely fall apart. I think it is *all* perfectly acceptable. Why?

It is my perspective that love and death are the things all humans have in common. They are the ultimate bonds between us all. It is grand to think of this in a planetary way, stepping far up for that 30,000 foot view of everything. When we look at the bigger picture, we can be a tiny bit kinder to our neighbors here on earth. That's my personal opinion, and my personal mission.

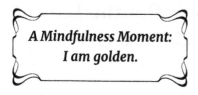

A Mindfulness Moment:
I am golden.

I believe we are but a blink of the eye and gone. We are an itty bitty speck of sparkling, shiny, gorgeous, glittery lint on the universe. Then, in heaven, or in another dimension, the energy world, etc., we have to carry on doing the soul work we have been given to do, or have chosen to do, or both. *What we think and what we do matters, a lot*, even in our tiny moments here on earth. Our essence lingers, weaving yet another golden thread in the majestic tapestry of the whole cosmos, and leaves a warm, vanilla-scented, love-filled trail after we are gone.

Becoming aware of this through the death of a loved one is a gift, really. It is nearly impossible to see so clearly during the blurry, teary, muddy, murky, messy time surrounding death though. If the death was sudden, brutal, or exceptionally tragic, it is my belief that God has major lessons for those left behind. The chance to grow exponentially is there if we want it, and then, if we go grab it.

As with all of our life challenges, when we apply conscious effort and hands-on, mindful work, the memory of death may not *always* be a source of pain, but may evolve into a loving memory, or a life lesson gained.

My Story: what you do matters

When I was eight years old, my maternal grandmother passed away of cancer. It was not sudden; there had been previous breast cancer that returned to claim the rest of her body. What I remember of that day was the family being in her house in Ohio, and the many relatives taking turns going into her bedroom to hold her hand, to speak their deep and endless love for her, to say, "See you later." I heard my grandmother laugh, loud, strong, and clear. It was as if these people's hearts healed her for a few moments.

I walked in gingerly when it was my turn and quietly placed my right ear to her heart, and said, "I love you Grandma Apple. Remember the time we laughed so hard at the dinner table that milk came out of my nose?" She smiled and put her hand on my hair. I quietly left the room, as it was one of the many other relatives' turns to be with her.

After Grandma Apple died, my mother thought it was important for me to go back into the bedroom and be with my grandmother again. At this point, it scared me shitless. I had never seen a dead person before, except on television shows. It was almost as if the person I pressed my head next to in caresses a few minutes beforehand was now a stranger. My mother, while being so gentle with me, led me into the room and made me hold my grandmother's hand. My mom, the firstborn of six children, bravely said, "Isn't she peaceful? Isn't she beautiful? Don't be afraid, honey. Grandma Apple is in heaven now. She's not in pain anymore. She's with Buube (great grandmother)."

The gift of connectedness my mom gave to me at that moment when I was afraid was an *aha* moment for me. Since then, I have always asked my relatives and friends who have passed on to send me advice, messages, and useful information for *my* future. I feel like their gifts do live on, absolutely. That is their legacy. They have answered my many questions right before I go to sleep, during that in between place of awake and asleep.

My own solution to the pain I suffered when my grandmother died was to begin cleaning and organizing. My need to make sense of something that seemed senseless was important to me. I needed to see a visible, positive result from the life I lived and the actions I took daily during that time of recovering and healing. I needed to clean. I emptied out my dresser drawers, scrubbed the interiors, placed toys and clothes that I no longer wanted in boxes or bags for donations, and continued until my room was beautiful and immaculate. It emerged as my new sanctuary. It was a new place of refuge and prayer for me, rather than a place to just play and sleep.

Over the years, I have continued to react to stress and chaos, and to loss and misunderstandings, by cleaning and organizing. It is something I can successfully control. With every repetitive swipe of the washcloth, I think things through, trying to make sense of everything. It reminds me of the movie *The Karate Kid*. When the student repeatedly waxed on and waxed off the master's car, he was in a sort of meditation. Afterwards things became clearer for his life's purpose. The same thing holds true for me.

More recently, one of my elder brothers passed away. My brother Danny perished from a fast acting, fatal pulmonary disease that has no definitive cause and no cure. Our entire family felt blindsided and lost. Once again, I found my solace in cleaning.

When I flew back to Pennsylvania for the funeral service, I stayed with my cousins in the home where I was born and raised. I practically begged them to allow me to clean the wooden floors before the memorial meal, which was to be held there. My emotions poured forth into the rags, and tears mingled with the lemon oil as I rubbed the wood shiny.

There. Done. It was late. I was tired. The funeral was the next day and we all needed to get some rest. My coping technique made me feel a tiny bit better.

Every stroke and swipe of the rag also allowed me to reflect back to a few days earlier in San Francisco, where I had a spiritual experience relating to my brother's soul beginning the transformation out of his body. I will explain further.

I was in my powder room on a typically chilly, foggy, San Francisco day in the late afternoon. All of the windows and doors were closed. I looked down at the floor, and right there in the center of the throw rug was a gorgeous brown and yellow butterfly. The butterfly flew up into my right palm and calmly stayed there. It did not flutter its wings at all. Immediately, instinctively, I knew it was Danny telling me that it was okay if I didn't come to Pennsylvania to visit him in the intensive care unit in his current state of illness. *He was visiting me.* He was telling me thank you for our loving relationship, years of shared laughter, our vacation together, and our life together as siblings. He was telling me that he was light as a butterfly now, assuring me that I was also going to be okay.

"Float like a butterfly, sting like a bee."
—Muhammad Ali

That's the quote that comes to my mind. A death sting for those of us left behind, but it is light for those going to the other side. That's the bittersweet moment I had. I took the butterfly outside after five minutes in my bathroom. I placed it on the back porch banister. The butterfly immediately *jumped (not flew)* onto my sweater sleeve and stayed there another 15 minutes. It got cold and dark as I continued to talk to Danny through the butterfly. (My kids were watching this exchange through the den window.) I then said goodbye and placed the butterfly down on the banister again, and slipped inside to warm up.

Side note: Danny wore a butterfly bow tie to work every day for years.

I believe spirits can morph and travel as we leave our bodies through higher meditative states, enlightenment, remote viewing, dreams, and death states. I had the same butterfly experience one time prior when a cousin passed away.

So, why am I telling you all this? Symbols in our lives hold deep meaning for individuals and tribes (families) through rituals and happenstance both. We look for meaning in the small every day experiences and the physical things involved, especially when dealing with the loss of a loved one. The movie ticket stubs that we find in a pants pocket are trash when we do laundry, but they become a treasure, a source of memory and reverence if the pants belonged to a loved one who has passed away.

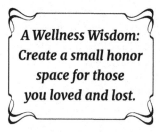

A Wellness Wisdom:
Create a small honor
space for those
you loved and lost.

I suggest folks place these things we come upon and revere into a small honor box. I am not suggesting we become pack rats and never get rid of the things that we no longer need or use for the sake of honoring the memory of a dead relative or friend. We must heal and move forward.

The difference between surviving and thriving after the loss of a loved one is whether or not one can honor, love, and eventually grow as a human being themselves for having known the other person (and not die themselves under the weight of the pain). It is a matter of baby steps.

First, and foremost, we must surround ourselves with love. Then we can build a support system. The support system may consist of religious or psychological groups, or friends and family members who instinctively know how we react in stressful situations. Please, please, please do not be afraid to say the words, "Help. I'm so sad, scared, lonely, and lost."

My father passed away just three months after my brother Danny. My dad was 93, in the late stages of Alzheimer's disease, and no longer recognized any loved ones. I had visited him a few weeks before he died. I rubbed his head, fed him chocolate chip cookies, and kissed his cheek a hundred times.

He thought I was a very nice police chief. When I told him I loved him, he kept saying back to me, "I love you ma'am." There was a flash of recognition in the hours I was there, a moment where he grinned widely, and the light in his eyes changed. I do think he knew who I was for just a moment. I cling to the hope and memory of that moment.

Of course, I have many great memories of my dad, but there were very few during the last six years of his life. Still, his passing was not earth shattering to me. He lived a long life. He was blessed to make it to 93. Perhaps all of my anguish and tears had been spent on my brother, and I just didn't have any heartache left. Maybe I had said goodbye a long time ago, when his memory faded. In any case, I felt very peaceful and very okay with my father's passing.

A Wellness Wisdom: Crying is essential for emotional expression and healing.

I don't know why we attempt to stop grief from arising. I suppose it is to put on a brave front or to make other people feel less uncomfortable. When that grief becomes inevitable, we must somehow process that grief. Healthy grieving is good and necessary. It is essential for mental and physical well being. I suggest that we do not suppress our grief. Suppressing grief is dangerous to the immune system too. Tears are cleansing, and they hit our reset button so we can regain the capacity to be happy once more. If we process the grief without much attention, it can become a much deeper sorrow. Grief may manifest itself in unexpected ways:[10]

- Grief can disrupt sleep. It may invade our dreams too.

- Grief can actually physically weaken the body.

- Suppressed grief can numb us in many ways: sexually, psychologically, and spiritually.

- Grief may make us feel empty.

Unattended sorrow narrows our path in life. There may be a lack of richness and fullness in all of the other emotions. In my opinion, we need to pause in our lives and attend to our feelings. Then we can do more than survive. We can actually thrive and go beyond normal, beyond neutral. We can become our superior selves.

There is no hierarchy in loss. When people talk about death, they seem to feel like there is a hierarchy around loss but there is none. I lost my brother, my father, my uncle, and two of my children's best friends within a year and a half.

Does that mean that I am higher on the *feeling sorry for myself* plane or that you should feel more sorry for me than someone else? Does the type of loss you suffer make you *one-up* me? "But you don't understand," people tell me. The point here is to have compassion, love and empathy at best and sympathy at the very least. We cannot put ourselves completely in other people's shoes because we have not 100% been in their shoes, nor will we ever be, but we are all connected. Communication creates connection creates community.

Normal Grieving Phases

Normal grieving has coping phases which include:

- Denial

- Anger

- Bargaining

- Depression

- Acceptance

There is no length of time for any of these stages, and one may enter and exit these phases many times until one is finished. It is an individual and unique process. These grieving phases are commonly observed in the behavior of terminally ill patients, but are in the normal ranges of behavior in those around the dying during the months before dying. After someone passes away, these feelings and thoughts also are in the normal ranges of those grieving.[11]

Denial

Denial is a defense mechanism that allows a person to cope for a little while. The person may change the subject when death is brought up. One in denial may not even wish to associate with others who want to help out in a loving and caring manner. One in denial may refuse to go to the memorial service or hospital, even in the case of a spouse or child. They may act bright and cheery as if nothing is out of the ordinary.

Anger

Anger is what typically replaces denial when one cannot live in the space of make-believe any longer. One asks, again and again, "Why?" The anger may be projected randomly towards anyone and everyone, and at random times as well. Then later on, one may feel guilt and shame surrounding their behavior. This doesn't help at all. It is reassuring to know that this theme is natural and acceptable.

If you are being attacked verbally by a terminally ill or grieving individual, understand that it is not really about you at all. Respect, accept, and understand that, please. It is hard not to take it personally, especially when anger is being directed towards you, but breathing deeply and counting to ten will help both parties get through the moment.

Bargaining

Bargaining is where one pleads with the Universe, with God, with All That Is.

Here is an example of bargaining: "If I do everything perfectly and according to your will, can You fix this or reverse this? I'll keep up my end of the bargain if You keep up Your end of the bargain, OK? Bring back my dead son. Turn back the hands of time. I'll never steal again if You bring back my dead son."

Depression

Depression may follow when a person is not given the answer he or she asked for during bargaining. There is a sense of loss. There may also be a loss of income surrounding death. One may need to take time off from work for visits to the hospital, and there may be a lack in one's ability to be productive at all while at work. The person who passed away may have contributed financially to the family's needs. This is a time when one feels so hopeless and insignificant in the world. (Journaling, nature, and support groups are exceptionally useful here.)

Acceptance

Acceptance comes with time. Acceptance comes with help from outside sources. Acceptance comes after working internally on the self, the soul, and the previous stages. Acceptance comes when we are too darned tired to fight with ourselves anymore, and so we peel back the outer layers of rotten cabbage leaves and reveal the shiny, dewy, inner layers waiting to be exposed, seen at a different angle or point of view. There's no more fear or despair. It has been replaced by a sense of *okay* or even contentment.

Davey and Don's Story: feeling abandoned and acting out

Two brothers, Davey and Don, lost their parents in an automobile accident when the children were eleven and thirteen. Davey was the older sibling. The kids were placed in a foster home together. The new foster parents were upbeat and positive in their outlook on life. They didn't believe in living in the past, however, so they didn't take the boys to grief therapy or counseling to deal with their loss. They weren't very religious either, so they didn't have a spiritual leader to turn to for the transitions and the boys' coping techniques. They did, however, take them on trips to see the world and learn about other cultures. The foster parents felt like this was a way to regain connectedness to others, and to see the value of the wide, wonderful world around them.

Just a year or so later, Davey and Don began partying after school with friends. They began getting high and sneaking alcohol. Their grades suffered the effects. They were trying to show the foster parents that they were independent and could do grown up things, like drinking and getting high. They desired attention, but couldn't say so out loud. They felt like their feelings were dismissed by the foster parents at the initial time of their grief. This was their way of kind of punishing the foster parents. They liked them because they were young and hip, but parenting boundaries and tough love were very much needed.

During the school year, several counselors and school psychologists in their middle and high school held interventions with the kids and their foster parents. They wanted to facilitate some movement with the unattended grief and repair the relationships between the boys and their new family before they were irreparable. Finding a new foster family would be nearly impossible.

Davey and Don did not intentionally make others suffer with their actions, but "suffering" was what everybody at this point was feeling. The boys didn't want to feel alone in their grief. The boys felt like they were drowning in their despair, and they believed that every adult they knew and loved would leave them at some point. They were mad that their parents had left them, even though it was not their parents' fault. They were grieving the lost relationship. They grieved the relationship they wished they had to build upon.

The counselors focused on what the boys' interests were, like painting and writing music. They used these arts to help the new family unit get their emotions out, so the self destructive behavior had a chance to possibly cease. The sessions had the whole family painting, writing lyrics, talking, shouting, singing, and crying together. When anger was shown, it was in a safe place. They were told to regularly make a bonfire in the backyard, to burn up the paintings and music they no longer wanted to keep; that is, the feelings they no longer harbored towards the world.

After several cathartic bonfires, Davey and Don were able to begin anew with the foster parents. Issues surrounding abandonment and death are never easy, whether intentional or accidental. We all deserve unconditional love, security, and a good foundation.

The counselors worked together developing a long term system of checking on the boys. Every Monday the boys would write down how they were generally coping with their world in a little notebook. On Friday, they would look at the notebook and note changes, good or bad. It only took a few minutes, and was a good way to self check their emotional state so things would not get out of control again. If they were feeling angry, frustrated or negative towards themselves or others, they were to go discuss their feelings with their foster parents. This was a method for the boys to grow into trusting adults again, and to know that they were loved and cared for. Being consistently aware of their emotional state, and discussing what was important to the boys' lives was paramount in their healing as a new type of family unit.

Because they were young, they involuntarily fell into, "I should have, I would have, and I could have." In each of their minds, "If only I had been ill that day, my parents would have stayed home, and then they wouldn't have had an auto accident." (There are so many involuntary scenarios that play out in one's mind in hindsight. These help to make sense of the senseless.)

Feeling helpless as kids eventually shifted into feeling powerful and creative as adult artists. Their art ultimately made them stronger during their healing years, and showed that they had much to contribute to the world. Davey and Don not only bounced back, the boys rebounded upwards and their artistic talents grew into abundances for many. They were well known artists in their city, held shows twice yearly, and created a program where they mentored other youth healing from the death of a loved one through art therapy.

A Wellness Wisdom: Guilt is self induced.

When we attend to our deeper selves, we do not lose ourselves. On the contrary, we find ourselves. We eventually heal, and become even more comfortable with who we are. Grief does not always disappear completely, but it can morph into something we can work with. There is a difference between letting go, and completely forgetting. When we heal with positive actions, we face our superior selves head on. We then can smile and nod *yes* at what we can become.

An Invitation: draw the pain away

Think about the loss of a loved one. Take crayons, paints, colored pencils, or any art tool and draw your feelings. It doesn't have to be images or objects that others can identify. It can be scribble-scrabble. Draw for as long as you like. Many of us haven't picked up a crayon since elementary school. It is very freeing, knowing that there is no judgment or grade attached to the art you are making. It is an outpouring of your heart. If the art is something you want to destroy afterwards, then do that.

Sometimes we feel like we do not deserve to have fun when we are grieving. We catch ourselves laughing and feel guilty. Our friend sees us putting on makeup and going on a date when they think it is too soon to be dating. There is a silent unappointed *committee. Fire the committee. Release the guilt.*

Living Beyond the Pain

We *can* live beyond what we think we are capable of. Just look at world records in sports, or the Olympics. As soon as we see a new world record in something, the next time that effort and accomplishment is blown out of the water by yet another athlete, we are in awe all over again. Impossible! How did they do that? The answer is they changed the language. When we change the language, we can change the mind. When we change the mind, we can change the belief system. When we change the belief system, we can change our reality.

When we come out of the fog of grief, we can think of the relationship we had with that person, the whole gamut. In my head it goes something like this, "I love you and you are woven into my history and prayers." The tapestry of one's humanity is in the people they meet and touch.

This works in surviving the death of a loved one too. Instead of telling yourself that you can't go on, that everything is forever doomed, tell yourself what you *can* do, right now. Do not deny your feelings, but tell yourself one small thing that you can do to survive today, right now. Remembering what the dying relative or friend embraced as he or she left earth can be a lesson for us. What he or she was able to completely let go of as they left earth can also be a life lesson for us. When we witness another's graceful exit to the other side, we may more fully understand what it is to be in a human body.

Experiencing the death of a loved one gives us the chance to reach for *our* higher power, to pray and meditate, *even if we never did it before.* If the language changes, everything can change. Reach out to those who you know have the time and energy to support you. Devote yourself to yourself. I believe that with time and self love, we can do more than survive. We can thrive.

Note to Those Supporting Those Grieving

Attentive listening is important at this time in the grieving person's life. Be wholly present and not distracted while the grieving person is pouring out his or her heart to you. If you are thinking of your 2:30p.m. tennis match, the grieving individual will intuitively know. Now is the time for your complete attention and acceptance, but be cautious with opinions. Your relationship may depend on this.

Conscious of it or not, we are all on a quest for answers. Death brings these questions to the forefront: Who am I really? What are the lessons of life? Why are we here?

What is love? What is true power? Can we ever be truly happy? And then, where do we begin to look for answers?

"Oh, I'm so inadequate — and I love myself!"
—Meg Ryan, actor

Most humans are riddled with fear of death and guilt over our relationship mistakes. I encourage you to reach for your higher power, whatever that is for you. Build a tribe of support in your family, community, faith, or counseling services. Surviving the death of a loved one is a defining moment where we are shaken to our core, and we may build a new foundation with some new truths. Being at the edge of our own death, or of someone close to us, we may finally find meaning through prayer, creativity, or meditation. We may *get it*. We may have a larger orb of energy around us. We can have a greater understanding of *everything*. And then it ripples outward towards everyone else.

The tough lessons of life and loss are facets of our human core spirit. When we accept the shifts, no matter how long or how much effort it takes, eventually we may become different people than we were before and shake the fall leaves off, so to speak. After grieving, bereavement counseling, community, connection, love, and self-care, our true colors may emerge, shine and we may reach our *Happy, Healthy Selves*.

Chapter Nine

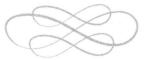

Silence as a Healer ~ Shut Up Already!

When I practice yoga, any kind of yoga, I must be silent. Being silent is really, really, *really* difficult for me. After all, I am a mama, a wife, a server, a writer, a workshop facilitator, a wellness coach, and a social butterfly. I have to communicate for my life's work, and I'm great at doing just that, all of the time! When I force myself to shut up, it is a struggle, and an exercise in discipline. I sooooooo need this.

Silence leads to great ideas, *aha* moments, divine inspiration being whispered to me on the winds, and a gentle sort of self-forgiveness. Silence is a healer.

Yoga forces me to be silent. My favorite kind of yoga is Bikram hot yoga. It is a ninety minute class of intense poses held for sixty seconds for the first set, and then thirty seconds for the second set. Did I mention that it is hot? The room is 105 degrees Fahrenheit to begin with, and gets hotter when more practitioners attend. We aren't allowed to speak in class, providing me with yet another layer of self discipline, besides the heat and movements themselves. My silence is a kind of meditation for me, even though the teacher is talking.

My mental clarity grows as my practice strengthens and my flexibility expands. With regularity, silence allows me to forgive myself for mistakes made and unkind thoughts that drift in daily. I even started to be less anal in other areas of my life!

The word *yoga* means union. It is specifically the union of body and mind. I think the breath is what unites the body and the mind in a yoga class. I imagine the breath is a thread slowly sewing the body and mind together through the stretches and compressions of the body work. It is also the union of the people in the room working together toward a common goal. Any time we have a group of people collectively focusing on one thing it is powerful, a collective consciousness. It is healing.

Does anybody remember Hands Across America? It was an event in the summer of 1985, where folks literally held hands *silently* for peace for a certain number of hours, all across the United States of America, a chain of hands and mindset. I was living in Washington, D.C. at that time. It was an amazing event to partake in, full of collective hope. Folks would come in and out of the chain as restroom, hunger, and diaper changing needs became apparent, but someone else would grasp the hand and keep the chain of world peace alive. Yes, ordinary people can do extraordinary things, together, with intention, silently, in connection, in community.

❦

An Invitation: personal forgiveness

Say out loud, "I don't enjoy _____ about myself."

Now breathe in deeply through the nose and as you exhale say the exact opposite statement, "I enjoy _____ about myself." Breathe in and out again, silent on the inhale and saying the positive words on the exhale.

Say, "I forgive myself for thinking negatively about myself, but it simply is not true."

With practice, even if you don't believe it at first, the repetition of changes in the language will yield changes in the mind. The belief will shift over time, probably more rapidly than you believe right now!

An Invitation: yoga

Most gyms and yoga studios have the first class available for free. If you are in a rural area, there are free classes on cable television, and DVDs to borrow from the library. It may sound hippy-trippy to do, but if a thoroughly modern, type A personality like me can attempt one class, so can you. Nobody cares if you do not know the moves or how deep you can go into each posture. They are too focused on their own practice. Enlist a friend to practice with you if you are shy or embarrassed about beginning. Remember, everybody is a beginner at something, all of the time. This tool in the wellness toolkit has literally helped me through many personal hardships and through everyday stress. I invite you to give it a shot.

Yoga is hard at first. Any stretching exercise (or any fitness program) is hard at first. Yield to the pain. There is a difference between discomfort and pain. We can live with a little discomfort and grow through the discomfort, but yield to the pain. That works in life as well as in yoga.

Warning: Sometimes when we go with a friend to a class, we will watch them to see how they are faring in the class. We will watch the people around us, and sometimes we may mentally leave our own journey in order to join theirs!

I am a victim of this above (**warning**) scenario. When I am behind a person who just won't listen to the teacher, or doesn't understand, part of me observes and wants so very much to whisper to them, "Feet together! Breathe through your nose! No water yet!" My frustration and desire to be a good neighbor and helper causes me to leave my yoga practice right then and there. I catch myself having to mentally pull back the reins, recommit to my own practice and to my own discipline, and leave them alone!

If my goal is to heal through the silence and the practice, then I must serve myself and myself only. How often do we get to do that during the rest of the day? Some teachers advise students to leave whatever is outside of the studio, outside of the studio. It will be there when we are done. The struggle is part of the story. It is not, however, the whole story.

"The right way is the hard way."
—Bikram Choudry

I have heard this saying so many times during my years of studying hot yoga. Usually the teachers are referring to very difficult poses. The yoga instructors say that the meaning behind the quote is that it is far more beneficial to the body to practice the poses with the correct technique a little bit the right way, even though it is hard to master. Do not cheat. Then as time goes on, when we gain strength and flexibility, we may push ourselves deeper and deeper into the poses. Then we may hold the poses longer and longer. Perhaps we may try one set of poses rather than two sets the first few weeks of our yoga practice. It took me almost three years to finally be able to balance on one foot while squatting cross-legged (toe stand). But when I did, oh, the party in my head was so awesome!

The poses that are the hardest to do are the ones we need the most. Life is like that too. The lessons in life that are the hardest to swallow are the ones we get the most out of. Life lessons and healing come in a variety of modalities, like *31 flavors*.

We are a work in progress in life outside of yoga and silence. "The right way is the hard way." This speaks to me in my everyday challenges, my work drama, and my trauma recovery as well. The gratification and satisfaction of figuring things out and rising above my troubles is so sweet! Think about how sweet a first sip of water tastes after a hard, long bike ride, or after a good crying session. The right way is the hard way (no matter what your smart phone tells you). Struggling through the hard parts of life builds strength and stamina for your *whole* life.

The Beginner's Mind

The beginner's mind: What is it? It is experiencing the activity as if doing it for the first time.

I have been practicing yoga off and on since I was fifteen years old, and more recently, consistently for several years. After a week of the flu and no yoga, I went back to class. What surprised me the most was not my lack of muscle tone or strength, but my new ability to feel like a beginner. It was as if I was hearing the words for the very first time. Different details and nuances of the instruction came forth for me. Even the instructor's voice sounded velvety and different. I was not just going through the motions. I was paying great attention to my intention and practice.

How can we embrace the beginner's mind? How are we to go back there? I think the best way to embrace the beginner's mind is to teach a child or a friend something that we are very skilled in. When we teach another the basics of any skill, we must imagine ourselves in their shoes and be empathetic at best, and sympathetic at the very least.

When we are silent, we can shake off the therapy session, the argument, or struggle we just went through. In order to be strong, happy, independent, and healed, I say we must add silence into our toolbox of healing techniques. Silence allows us to reorganize, re-energize, process, and integrate the challenges we are going through.

Another way I embrace silence is to go outside for a walk, hike, or run in nature. Do not underestimate the power of the sun, moon, and wind to clear the mind of negativity. When I walk in the woods or hike a mountainside, I increase oxygen consumption, my immune system improves, and I utilize all five senses! If I'm silent on my walks or runs, I allow the creativity to flow even more and I solve all of the world's problems, mine included. While I was jogging on the beach and silently watching the ocean waves crashing upon the San Francisco shores, I received the name of my website and brand, *Superior Self*. Between the sweat, the silence, and the feel-good hormones, creativity was born. I stopped the world long enough to listen to the universe for answers.

An Invitation: walk outside in silence

Go outside in a grassy or tree-filled area for a walk or jog for at least thirty minutes. Walk slowly, briskly, or jog. The speed does not matter. It will steady the mind, clear the angst, and add oxygen to the body. Walking outside releases feel-good hormones called endorphins. These hormones make us feel like everything is all right with the world, at least for a little while. The more often and longer we go out and play in nature, the greater the benefits and the longer they last.

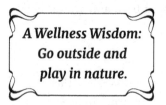

A Wellness Wisdom:
Go outside and
play in nature.

Pay attention to your breath. Try to hear the inhalation and exhalation through your nose. When we simplify our whole, complicated life down to a breath, we can momentarily let go of some things.

We can finally relax our tense shoulders, our tight jaws, our million-miles-a-minute minds. Real healing can begin.

In Japan, there is a nature prescription called shinrin-yoku. Shinrin-yoku consists of day trips to the forest, also called forest bathing. Walking silently in nature connects us to a bigger picture. The benefits of forest bathing include positive neuropsychological effects on the nervous system. The hormone adiponectin is also increased. A lower level of adiponectin is linked with obesity and conditions related to obesity. Studies have shown that forest bathing reduces stress, anxiety, depression, and sleep problems.[12] Spending time in nature builds the immune system as well. Some doctors in Japan literally write a prescription for shinrin-yoku on prescription pads to overworked and over stressed patients![13]

Hillary and Mickey's Story: a silent cry for help

Hillary was a busy, working mom of three kids, whose ages ranged from three to ten. In order to support their family, she and her husband, Mickey, worked opposite hours. They saved on childcare costs that way. Unfortunately, it didn't leave them much time together as a family, and nearly no time together as a couple.

After three years with no vacation, the woman was at her wit's end. She loved every part of her life, but it was making her exhausted, and she missed her dear partner of fifteen years, even though they were living in the same house. Hillary came across a website one night when she was surfing the internet, dreaming of a getaway. It was a gorgeous meditation center in the wilderness, and it was free! All they had to do was work in the kitchen or farm a few hours a day for payment. It also required complete silence.

Without hesitation, she signed up for the weeklong retreat for the two of them. When she told her husband, Mickey stated that a meditation retreat was not what he had in mind for a vacation. Who was going to take care of the kids? They had never meditated before, never farmed before, and had never left their children with relatives before. (Oh, did I mention it was a silent retreat? They had never done that before either.)

Following her instincts, Hillary knew that this just had to happen or she would go nuts from the stress and possibly ruin the family dynamics in the process. Luckily, they convinced the kids' favorite aunt to stay with them, and off they went.

The first day was the hardest, and to ensure silence, everyone slept in beds with curtains around them, dorm style. It helped with accountability. Hillary and Mickey fidgeted physically like children the first half of the day, but by dinner time on the first day they were actually seeing the benefits of being quiet, meditating, and getting out in nature together.

After the retreat, they were refreshed, and the answers to their busy-ness appeared in the silence. Mickey decided to work less hours because his job paid lower wages than Hillary's. They decided to arrange to take the same work days off, and one night each week would be date night, now that they saw how the children had survived without them (just fine) for the week. The children bonded with their favorite aunt even more, and the kids created special memories of their own while Mommy and Daddy were away.

Healing through silence shows that we have the ability to triumph despite tragedy, and we can reach victory despite everyday stressful events as well. Let's face it. Most of us need to shut the heck up more often than we like to admit, but we never thought of the quiet as medicine, as therapy, as a way to receive answers from...

Being mindful and present is difficult, especially since we are very attached to our electronic devices. When I ask my kids if they are enjoying their dinner and whether they want more food, the answer is, "I'm good." I get so frustrated with that answer, and we have had family discussions about this. I ask them a yes or no question, not a good or bad judgment question. I know they are *good*, fine, and sweet. I am also guilty of not paying attention to conversations at times.

I do not want to engage in a huge debate about cell phones and screen time here, but I do want to say that silence is another important restorative practice to pull out of the toolbox. Unplugging, getting regular time off of autopilot, and getting outside to nature will be beneficial for the body, brain, emotions, and relationships. It will be healthful whether you are in tip-top shape or recovering from surgery, cancer, depression or loss. It is helpful whether you are silent *with or without* a friend next to you. Go twice in one day if you must photograph the breathtakingly beautiful area; one time with the device and one time without. It does a body good!

Meditation as a Recovery Tool

Meditation has been used in mindfulness based therapeutic psychotherapy for many years, with favorable outcomes in anxiety, depression, addictions and hormonal disorders.

Meditation is silent. Meditation is a practice that is for many of us a difficult challenge to attempt. It is another type of discipline. We use the word discipline in our society frequently meaning consequences or punishment. Why do I have to do something so hard, so punishing in order to help me out with my other daily challenges?

What exactly *is* meditation? A simple answer for a non-religious person is: focusing on the breath while allowing the thoughts in your mind to pass through without judgment. Stop looking so hard for something that is missing and *relaaaaax*. Stop the insanity. If a thought won't stop bugging you, allow it in, but say to it, "You gotta pay rent to stay." Then allow it to flow through you. How?

Here is how I am able to stop the busy-ness for just a few minutes of freedom, enough to create true healing.

I practice a style of meditation I thought up a couple of years ago, for just a couple of minutes a day, after yoga. That's all the "regular" meditation I can handle. (Yoga is a moving meditation.) Sometimes I do this before work too, in my car. It sets me up for a great day or night.

An Invitation: number meditation

Close your eyes and I think of the number 1. It could be a fat one, a skinny 1, or a puffy clouded 1, like on the TV show, *Sesame Street*. Inhale and exhale slowly and think of 1, 1, 1. Then think of the digit 2, 2, 2, in the same fashion. You don't have to think of them 3 times. You can stretch out the digits by lengthening out the word very slowly in your head. If a thought or an errand enters your head, and they will, do not judge yourself. Just think, "Okay, what number am I on?" Go back to the number. Then, when you get to number 10, go back to 9, 8, 7, and so forth. When you get down to number 1 go up to number 2 again. To me, the cycle feels like an infinity symbol. Do this up and down two times and it will take a few minutes. After a few months you may want to stretch out your vacation time.

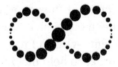

Massage for Silent Therapeutic Touch

I enjoy getting massages. My evenings as a server leave my shoulder muscles knotted up sometimes. I exercise a lot too. I want and need a deep tissue massage to get the tightness out and relax me from head to toe. One time, as my regular massage therapist worked on my body, I peeked at him and saw his eyes were closed. He was purposefully taking away one of his own senses, sight, and enhancing the sense of touch, silently feeling where I needed healing and work.

People often think of massage as a luxury. It is a luxurious feeling, for sure, but it is a necessary form of touch and does not have to be expensive. Touch is free and healing both mentally and physically. Ask a friend or loved one to massage you. This tool in the wellness toolkit is one of my favorites for grownup girlfriends' sleepover parties.

When I gave birth to my son, Golden, the delivery room staff kept saying to my husband and me to stay nude, under the covers, as much as we could during the first few months, and have skin to skin contact with the infant. They told us the baby needed our loving touch for survival and to thrive. We are tactile beings. Among mammals in the animal kingdom, it has been observed that newborns die without skin-to-skin contact, even if fed and kept warm. Skillfully manipulating and stimulating all of your skin, muscles, nerves, connective tissues, and joints through massage has a positive effect on the human body.

Massage has been shown to reduce anxiety and depression, and help with cancer patients' pain management. Giving compassionate attention through silent touch to chronically ill patients and senior citizens at senior homes has improved health markers overall. This is preventive health care and healing health care.

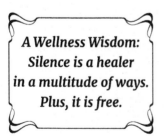

A Wellness Wisdom:
Silence is a healer
in a multitude of ways.
Plus, it is free.

Simply put, massage feels good, releases feel-good hormones throughout the body, is a silent healer, and allows its physiological and psychological benefits to work together. How much is that worth to you?

Small silent celebrations of the body and human spirit can enhance healing from stress, anxiety and chronic illness. Our point of view when beginning the simple tasks makes the difference. Here are some examples of normal tasks that can be silent healers:

- Painting our nails
- Painting a picture
- Writing a letter or card by hand
- Lighting a candle
- Praying
- Washing the dishes

- Folding laundry
- Spritzing on perfume or applying lotion
- Putting makeup on
- Lighting incense
- Taking a bath or shower

When we make small positive choices we are living our life positively. Dedicating silent moments is a wonderful addition to the wellness toolkit.

In the modalities of using silence as a healer we can once again find help from the three words **fuel, focus, and foundation**:

- **Fuel** is the slow and steady breath that accompanies the silent activity we embark on for coping and assisting in healing and recovery.

- **Focus** is the goal of total disconnect from our busy lives, the to-do list, the electronics, the tv, radio, media, etc. for just a little while. You are to be selfish, to dedicate yourself to yourself.

- **Foundation** is a deep grounding that occurs when you participate in consistent, silent self-care. You will emerge a *Happy, Healthy You.*

Chapter Ten

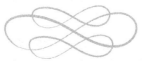

Compassion and Imagination to the Rescue ~ Tap Into Your Creativity

What is compassion? It is basically kindness, helpfulness, and supportiveness. I receive and give compassion every day, and it gives me an energy return that can't quite be described with words. When I am tending to another's needs in that very caring way, it lifts everybody in the situation upwards and outwards. It is also contagious. Have you ever put a quarter in another person's meter (on purpose)? Have you ever bought coffee for the person behind you in line at the coffee house, and quietly exited the shop? Those are examples of random acts of kindness that show compassion for strangers. Once you receive it, you usually want to do the same for others. Paying it forward can be really fun too.

My Story: compassion found in a cookie

After yoga one afternoon I was walking to my car quickly to get to work on time. Two men were rapidly walking towards me holding white Styrofoam bowls. As we passed each other we both slowed a little to gesture a hello with our eyes. I leaned a little too far forward to see what was in their bowls, and with all of my yoga bags, mat, wet towels, extra clothes, etc., made quite a spectacle of myself, nearly falling into them. One gentleman smiled and extended his hand with a bowl of macaroon cookie sandwiches stuffed with ice cream and gestured for me to take one. With his other hand he steadied my balance by grabbing my arm.

This silent gesture of offering a stranger a cookie and helping me keep my balance all at the same time was a moment of love and compassion that I'll never forget. A small act of compassion is not unnoticed. I can take that seed and plant it and water it. I can nurture it. You can too.

Love is the one thing that defies the laws of math. When you give it away freely, you gain more and more of it.

We can use compassion as a tool to heal during painful times and to help others grow in their times of need. General feelings of niceness can pervade the air, and despite it sounding rather Stepford Wife-like, everybody does like nice. If they carve on my gravestone, "She was nice," well, that's a beautiful statement about the sort of life I lived. That's good enough for me.

Imagination is the ability of the mind to be creative and resourceful, a spark of nothing becomes something by sheer thought. The ideas and images are formed by concepts not actually in our physical world. For example, I can see the table in the room, it is wood, and it is a shade of caramel brown. As I move closer to the table, I notice the grains of wood, the darker lines reminding me of a stream in a river moving rapidly in the rainy season. I hear the gurgle of the water as it splashes and changes direction over sharp rocks and worn down soft river rocks.

Compassion comes in many forms. We may close our eyes and imagine somebody acting in a kind, loving way (even if they aren't very kind in reality). We can wake up in the morning, and in the moments before we jump out of bed, imagine the day going exactly as we wish. These are examples of compassionate imagery. We can even use our imagination to put a positive spin on a bad memory. *Change the ending with our imagination.* This is another technique in the wellness toolkit that won't cost a dime and won't let us down.

Changing the outcome of a past misfortune with our imagination is also a way to actually change the chemistry in our brains. The feel-good hormones are released in the process. Using compassionate imagery creates a safe place within our body, a new place: the brain. Our imagination is endless, and it *is* under our control, so why not do something wonderful for ourselves?

Sometimes my children and I will start a game of street tag in a busy urban area of San Francisco. We start with just each other, and say, "Tag! You're it!" Then they must tag a stranger with the same words. They seek out someone who looks open and friendly. They must use their instincts. In the past, a whole block or two of San Francisco participated, and smiles lit up the streets! This was all due to a planned, compassionate, imaginative game! We imagined how the end would turn out, and we learned how to read people in the process. New connections are made and fear of the unknown dissipates. A sense of playfulness provides us with opportunities to use compassionate imagery!

Scent Creates Healing Imagery: therapy with candles, essential oils, and incense

When we have loving memories associated with certain smells, the compassionate imagery can be made that much stronger. When I feel out of sorts, have a bad day at work, or have an argument with a friend, I light a pumpkin spice, vanilla, or maple scented candle. Some days I light traditional Indian incense or Thai temple incense. Sometimes I go for the essential oil diffuser. I close my eyes, inhale the comforting scent, and clench my fists as tightly as I can for ten seconds. Then I go limp.

When I release my clenched fists, the anxiety is replaced (usually) with the memory of baking alongside my mother as a child. The warm oven heated me to my very core. The memories flood back of the radio blaring on the counter, with us chatting above the noise of the radio, or singing along as we prepared delicious treats to be gobbled up later, with the extras boxed up for the freezer. I remember the flour flying, and the mess not being judged, because we were *creating*. We were creating something with our hands together, she would place hers on top of mine, gently guiding my fingers as to the shaping and rolling of each pastry, making sure to lock the corners so the filling would not ooze out in the hot oven while baking.

This usually works for me, and my stress fades. I'm able to put things into perspective. Then I'm able to rehash my day and imagine a new solution to my negative feelings or to experiences that linger. I light different candles as my mood and the seasons change. I use scent to honor and reflect personal milestones.

Essential oils have been used for thousands of years. They have been used for physical ailments, stress, anxiety, and to make the space one is in have a calming or invigorating effect. Essential oils are used in personal care and for household cleaning. Our body understands natural. Our body knows what to do with natural. Natural understands natural.

> **A Mindfulness Moment:** **I'm listening to the ancient wisdoms of my ancestors whispering to me daily.**

Essential oils are plant based, so the old saying by Hippocrates, "Let food be thy medicine, and medicine be thy food" holds true in essential oil use as well. If we think of the origins of modern medicines, chemical copies are a pharmaceutical attempt to recreate the medicines that nature provides, without making them extinct. It is also easier and faster for pharmaceutical companies to chemically combine the separate parts in a lab instead of sending their teams out into the wild to gather for prolonged periods of time.

I am not against modern medicine. I love my ibuprofen, my cold medicines, and my prescriptions *when I cannot solve the issue by myself with food, massage, essential oils, or movement.* Sometimes we need a quick fix so we can go on being super human with our *busy-ness.*

I try to set the stage for prevention and minor personal issues with natural methods. Essential oils are part of my regime. They have been mentioned throughout history in every ancient book from the Bhagavad Gita, to the Bible, and the Koran. My friend and coworker Abji told me for years that he read and followed the plant based medical advice in the Koran, especially where sage, camphor, lemon, myrrh, cinnamon, cloves, thyme, sweet marjoram and honey were mentioned. Abji was reading and interpreting the Koran closely and went to his mosque weekly.

We use essential oils in three ways: in the air, on the skin, or ingesting them by mouth.

When using them in the air, I use a diffuser by putting water in the top chamber cup, and then putting 10-20 drops in the water. Then in the area below the cup I light a tea candle. Within minutes the room ambiance changes.

If using oils on the skin, which is our largest organ, we can absorb their benefits right through the skin immediately. It may take some time before the full benefits from essential oils are realized because it takes a while to circulate throughout the whole body. An essential oil may be used alone if the oil is mild in nature, or it may be used with carrier oils if the essential oil will cause skin to burn or blister. I like inexpensive grape seed oil as an unscented carrier. Grape seed oil also has small enough molecules to be absorbed by the skin. In my experience I have not had grape seed oil cause pimples or acne for my clients or for me. Other carrier oils that are safe to use are jojoba oil or almond oil. You may use coconut or shea butter, but be aware that these oils will turn solid at room temperature. They are great for making body butters. Personally, I use coconut and shea butters on my face every day.

If using in an oral application, I suggest making them into a hot tea by adding a few drops of essential oil to a mug of boiling water.

We may use essential oils alone or in combination with each other.

How are essential oils made? They are extracted by steaming the plants and skimming the oil off the top of the water. It takes a lot of the original plant to make just a little vial of essential oil. Because of that, it is super concentrated and effective. I compare it to juicing. I use about 40 pounds of green vegetables to make one gallon of green juice.

Quality essential oils are always food grade and therapeutic. Food grade means that whether we add the oil to our recipe for eating or not, it can be ingested without causing harm. An example is lemon essential oil or zest added to lemon curd. Therapeutic means it is for helping our body in some way. Some people cannot handle the intense aroma. I have had folks leave the library workshops because they had sensitivity to strong smells. Remember, everyone is responding to the myriad of tools in the toolkit here in an individual and unique manner. The goal is to end up a *Happy, Healthy You.*

Please seek out books and websites on oils and their therapeutic uses. Here are a few essential oils and their uses:

- Lemon oil or other citrus: for mental clarity and appetite suppression. I put essential oils of citrus in hot water, along with lemon juice for a drink when I am hungry. This can help us ascertain if we are really hungry, or just emotionally or socially hungry. Lemon oil is great for studying and learning.

I put lemon or citrus oil in a diffuser when doing research for my books. Lemon and citrus oils help cleanse the liver and calm the stomach, even though they smell and taste sour and acidic. Lemon in general creates an alkaline environment in the body. The lemon is acidic, but the stomach produces digestive enzymes to cool down those acids and therefore balance out the body. I also use citrus oils mixed with carrier oils for polishing my wood furniture. Lemon is also commonly used for sore throats.

- Lavender oil: most commonly used for sleep and relaxation. It also improves the mood. We can put some drops in the bath, on the pillow, or directly on the skin. If it is used on burns with carrier oils, it speeds healing. It is also good for itchy bug bites.

- Tea tree oil: good for acne and dandruff. Mix with honey for a facial mask. Put on foot fungus, cuts, wounds, and eczema rashes. Tea tree oil is good for killing mold and mildew in the house. I mix it with water or vinegar as a cleanser on my countertops. Then I burn a different, better smelling essential oil in a diffuser afterwards to make the air smell less sour from the vinegar.

- Peppermint and Spearmint oil: good for soothing the stomach when in pain, diarrhea, and bad breath. This is why gum often has peppermint oil in it. Peppermint aids the colon in digestion as well. In the Middle East and Africa, peppermint tea is offered after a meal rather than coffee. When I was in Turkey and Egypt every little rug shop or textile store offered me mint tea, and it is considered rude not to accept the kind gesture. I like to shop. What they didn't offer was a restroom (This became a problem for me). A few drops rubbed on the temples are good for headaches. When massaged on the chest, it helps with allergies and colds.

- Frankincense oil: this is the most common oil found in historical texts. It has been used in the healing of scars, in alternative cancer therapies, and for colon issues. Because of its healing properties, some high end anti-aging products use frankincense. This is the tip of the iceberg. If you are interested in the clinical data related to cancer and chronic diseases aided by essential oil therapy go to www.pubmed.org to find studies on essential oils and diseases.

- Rose oil: used as an anti-inflammatory. Rose oil may be used on the skin or in baking. There is a Moroccan restaurant in San Francisco that my family frequents and they use rose oil, orange oil, and lemon oil in their cooking. Sometimes rose oil is mixed with geranium oil and lavender oil. I mix them freely with carrier oils or with a saturated fat like coconut oil, cacao butter, or shea butter for a facial and body moisturizer. Geranium oil has been observed to balance the hormones in the body, especially during menopause.

- Energy oils: the most common essential oils for physical energy and mental stamina are rosemary oil, citrus (mentioned earlier), and cinnamon oil. Be careful about using cinnamon oil on skin without a diffuser. I took a bath in it once and had tiny blisters all over my body and face for three days. This is a testament to how concentrated it is. Rosemary and sage oils combined have been found to physically stimulate hair growth at the follicles. Now that is good energy.

- Fragrance Oils: other scented fragrance oils that are not essential oils may stimulate energy, but only use them in a diffuser, because they are not therapeutic and they are not food grade. Read your labels and ask questions of the shop staff where you purchase your essential oils.

This essential oil list is just the beginning of seeing scent as another tool in the wellness toolkit. It is another way to connect with our past, connect with others, and use imagination on the journey, rising up like a phoenix from the ashes.

When we use scent now to link to our past, perhaps we can recall good feelings. We can also use scent as a way to solve a current stressful situation by injecting the positive feelings and scent from our past into the current challenge. For example, for me, aromas of vanilla, cinnamon, sugar, and butter immediately recall baking with my mother early in the morning during winter break. The music was on the radio, the oven was warming up the kitchen, the snow was sparkling outside, and we were making something together, Hungarian pastries, as well as memories. Now, when I think about her current situation, living in hospice, with kidney failure and Alzheimer's, it stresses me out. She is so far away from me and I can't fix this. So, to alleviate my stress, I light a scented candle or diffuse essential oils of vanilla, cinnamon, orange, or pumpkin. I really do feel better because of the memories associated with those smells. It enhances the good feelings even more if I play music from my childhood.

An Invitation: scent exercise

Buy incense, candles, or essential oils that remind you of your favorite childhood memories. Light one and sit down nearby. Stare at the flame for sixty seconds. This will seem like an eternity. Inhale and exhale slowly through your nose, taking in the scent. Now close your eyes and recall the events surrounding this scent from your childhood. Why was this scent chosen? What in particular made the activity so special for you? Is there a way to recreate an activity with someone you love based around this scent or around the memory?

After a few minutes, go over the day. Was there a struggle you encountered? Does it seem so difficult or unfixable now? How might you look at the challenge with a different perspective? Does the good memory from your childhood flavor your approach now? If not, light another candle. Do the same work with this scent.

Summer's Story: honoring being different

Summer was an introvert from a very young age. She felt like she didn't fit in with the other kids in her neighborhood. Summer was very long and lanky when compared with other children at her elementary school. In the school class photos, she was the one in the back row, always next to the teacher, both because of her height and her comfort zone. Summer was more comfortable talking to adults than to kids her own age. She chose to go to the library rather than going to the playground at recess. She was often whispered about and teased a bit; it stayed just on the safe side of what we would call bullying. She tried to ignore it most of the time. Other times she tattled on them to her teacher.

Summer's parents supported her personality and character all the way. They felt she was an old soul. Summer was attracted to bugs, unlike other little girls in her elementary school. Her library hours were spent on reading everything she could about insects, both in fiction and in non-fiction works. At age eight, she told her parents that she wanted to try cooking bugs and eating them to see what they tasted like. Her parents agreed to this, but only if it was a whole family experience. They did the research on bug-eating cultures at the local library together. Rather than freak out or ostracize her choices, unusual as they were, they embraced the whole person. This compassionate way of dealing with an unusual child with creative and different tastes nurtured a strong, independent, and fearless childhood.

As an adult, Summer became a research scientist at a prestigious university in the field of entomology (the study of insects). When I met her, and we chatted about her seemingly awkward childhood, she told me that the library had saved her. The library was her closest friend growing up. Books never made fun of her for being quiet, never judged her for her choices or for the way she looked, and always gave her the gift of knowledge.

It was particularly important to Summer to tell me that the children's room in any library held a sort of magic for her. It became her safe place, a second home. Even the smell of the aged, wooden children's furniture was like an old friend greeting her each time she entered. It was her refuge, her sanctuary.

During our talks, Summer emphasized that children's books provided a simpler way to solve life's complicated problems. Children's books break down problems to the very basic elements. Children's books give a sense of ethics. They provide examples of the most important lessons in life. They share successes and victories over seemingly impossible obstacles. Kids' books give stories of hope, and stories of overcoming something difficult with grace. Summer said that she thinks people of all ages should spend time in the children's section of the library every week. The world would be a much better place if everybody did just that.

An Invitation: spend an hour in the children's area of the library (often!)

Go to your public library and make a beeline to the children's area. Look around at the books displayed on the top of the shelves. These are the ones that the librarian recommends for young readers. Choose one that speaks to you instantly, but you don't know why. Sit down and read it. Spend some time in silence learning from the lessons within the books. (Silence is a healing theme that repeats itself in many other exercises throughout this book.)

Contemplate how you may use these lessons for your own life's problems, and how to utilize them to heal from your own drama or trauma. Choose children's books that speak directly to your problems. Enlist the help of the librarian if you need to. This is your time to devote to you.

As my children got older and began to read long children's novels, I read right along with them. I often exclaim how amazing it is that children's novels have become my favorite fiction to read. I honestly have all but abandoned adult fiction in favor of children's fiction. The messages and universal themes of strength, dignity, doing the right thing, and positive outcomes continue to leave an indelible mark upon my soul.

When I ask people what their favorite childhood books are, they have immediate recall, their eyes shine, they smile, their breath quickens with excitement, and they share without hesitation. When I ask people what their favorite book is now, their eyes roll up to the ceiling in contemplation, there is a great pause, and it takes time to think of the answer. Usually there is much less enthusiasm too. It makes perfect sense to me, then, that many favorite childhood books are made into films that become blockbusters for a generation (*Harry Potter* or *The Hunger Games*, anybody?).

Films often take us on a journey away from our suffering, if only for a little while. Watching movies can be imagination therapy too. I often seek out films with the same types of conflicts and struggles that I am going through, either in order to see an outcome I desire or to witness a different point of view.

When we use imagination and compassion associated with love and kindness, we can be more generous with ourselves and more forgiving of others. Sometimes we just need a little reminder of how good things can be. Going into the world of children's books or films (and losing ourselves in the stories) takes us out of our miserable moments. We can disappear for a little while. This is a sort of meditation too.

Compassion and imagination are rescuers for when we feel dead inside. When we have life challenges and feel like the only place where we were truly free, where we were truly wholly ourselves, is ripped away from us, it feels devastating. Do not despair, though. Our sense of self and hope can be restored over time with purposeful compassion and intentional imagination.

Part of our life's journey is asking the questions, "Why me? Why now? Why does this anger and frustration well up at the most inopportune moments? Why don't I easily and swiftly have an answer? Why can't I work everything out in my head, like so and so did?" Comparing our own lives to others' is normal, yet can take us on a downward spiral of thinking of about if we are *good enough*. Grab a tool from the wellness toolkit instead.

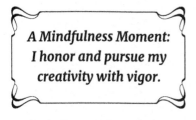

A Mindfulness Moment: I honor and pursue my creativity with vigor.

I encourage you to suspend your own (negative) belief system for a little while. Take time to receive and give compassion without regard to the outcome. The outcome will be good, believe me. I ask you to go into the world of make-believe with wild abandon. Afterwards, when the fork in the road presents itself (again and again), and a decision must be made, you will calmly and confidently choose the path that will serve you, and serve the world around you. Know it. Feel it. Believe it. I already see you grinning from ear to ear, a *Happy, Healthy You.*

Chapter Eleven

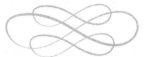

Epigenetics ~ Shifts in Potential

Why is it that the human condition allows us to succinctly remember every minute detail of when things go wrong in our lives?

For example, we may be having the best summer of our childhood, but the first thing that pops into our head when we think back to that summer is the moment we bit into a water bug, right in the center of our ice cream cone, thinking it was a praline pecan. We acknowledge, but downplay the rest of the summer's events: the endless nights of chasing fireflies, the movies watched in the park, the hikes with friends looking for fossils.

As a server for almost twenty years, I have had countless positive serving experiences, where the guests left happy, and said I contributed to their memories of San Francisco. Unfortunately, what rapidly comes to mind when thinking back over my serving career is the one woman who insisted that the kitchen didn't put the chicken in her chicken Caesar salad. She said that it was *my* fault, and that I was racist and didn't give her the chicken because she was African American. (For the record, she and her daughter ate the chicken; she just wanted more for free. Oh, did I mention my husband and children are African American?)

Perhaps remembering the horrible stuff prepares us for a swifter, alternative reaction in case we are faced with the same scenario again. We will survive the trauma and drama more rapidly the next time around, or develop ways to avoid it altogether. Does this go back to the time of the cave man? Are we hard wired and genetically coded to remember the yucky moments in order to protect our species for the future? Science says we do have a cellular memory.[14]

And this brings us to the title of this chapter, epigenetics. To better understand epigenetics, let us look at the word genetics.

Genetics in the study of our DNA, our inherited codes, and our likelihood to have similar looks, tastes, talents, and personality styles to our parents, grandparents, and further ancestors. I liken it to a pair of pants that was made in the factory with a sharp, apparent front crease, built in to the fabric. The whole shipment was created that way because of the factory settings. When we buy those pants at the store, we pretty much know what we are getting. The crease will be there for the life of the pants, wash after wash.

Epigenetics are the studies of when a consistent, repetitious change in the environment can have long lasting effects on a person, their kids, their kids' kids, etc. The effects can last generations after the first person was affected. The normal pattern of the genetic code is not enough to explain all that is going on within a family's lineage.[15]

I liken it to the creative kid who decides he isn't into a sharp crease in his pants, but his mom got them on clearance, so he can't return them. So, what does the kid do? The kid adds his own flair. He irons those pants flat every time he washes them. He distresses them with a small blade and tweezers, adding fashionable tears. He begins to make it his own. He embroiders on it and draws on it with fabric paint. And after a while, those pants are uniquely his, and anybody who looks at the pants a few months later would never know they were the permanently creased pants his mother got on sale. Years later, the kid is a grown up. From years of adding his own flair to pants, he creates his own factory line of non-creased, distressed pants. Of course, that's what his community expects from him *now*. And so it is with epigenetics.

Our food intake, our environment, our attitudes, and our daily experiences can change the very way our genes behave in future generations. Epigenetics is the marrying of nature and nurture.

Epigenetics have an impact on human health. Poor nutrition in one generation can have an impact on future generations. Data from the European famines during World War II support this idea.[16] Malnourished women who were pregnant at that time gave birth to more fragile babies. Even if the babies had plenty of nutritious food right after infancy, and continued to have it for the remainder of their lives, they were more prone to ailments related to malnutrition. Even the generation after the first shift was affected in a negative way. They too, were more prone to diseases of malnourishment, regardless of their nutritional intake.

The opposite results may also be true. If we are living in a society with an obesity epidemic (like now), our children's children may have tendencies to acquire type II diabetes more easily. In mouse experiments regarding obesity, it was found that the metabolism was affected in the generation following the initial obesity.[17] They also had a broken metabolism, and the liver composition was modified in multiple generations.

Children of mothers who suffered from Post Traumatic Stress Disorder as a result of the Holocaust were more inclined to develop PTSD in their lifetime, even though they had no direct experience of the Holocaust. This is a clear cut example of epigenetics at work. The same kind of experiences have been seen after the tragedy of 9/11. Mothers who were pregnant at that time gave birth to babies who now have reported more anxiety, stress, and PTSD symptoms than other children born after this era.

So, what does this all have to do with me? What do epigenetics have to do with me dealing with my stress and problems? How can this information help me become my superior self?

When we have a family history of alcoholism, depression, anger management issues, etc., we can easily say to others that we are struggling with these same challenges because it runs in the family (genetics).

These genetic predispositions do *not* have to be our crystal ball, our only insight into the future. With our big brains, knowledge, and new tools at our side, we can create our best expressions of ourselves. That is how epigenetics works. Our basic DNA doesn't change, but through our repeated choices, we can change who we are. We can reach our highest gene potential when we feed ourselves with mind-body-spirit food.

As I said before, it begins with a deep desire. What do you want? What do you want your legacy to be when you leave this world? Your fingerprint is yours only. It is unique. Press upon the earth your special imprint.

How we act, react, eat, sleep, work, love, and play creates our human experience and our human health. If I am in a generation that is predisposed to obesity (which I am), I can easily live up to those genetic expectations. Or, through a conscious, mindful effort to eat real, whole, unprocessed foods, exercise daily, meditate, sleep, and play, I can shift the hormones that want to keep me fat and unhealthy. With long term efforts, I can change my genetic expression and become a new example of what my template can be. If I choose the most nutrient dense options long enough, I may keep my children and grandchildren from easily becoming obese even before they are born.

Does this make sense?

We are partners with our bodies and minds. We have a huge responsibility to future generations. Let's not mess it up. Epigenetics works for mental disorders and stress related issues too, like perfectionism, type A personalities, anorexia, depression, alcoholism, etc.

Joshua's Story: a professional partier

Joshua did not come from a family of alcoholics. Joshua became a partier during his college years, and then continued his heavy drinking habit into his professional life.

When Joshua eventually found a life partner, they got pregnant with their first child right away, about three months into their marriage. Sarah, his wife, was not a heavy drinker. She had champagne on New Year's Eve, her birthday, and at others' weddings. Sarah didn't come from a family with a history of alcoholism either.

Their first child was born with a low birth weight and had some symptoms of infants who come from mothers who drank heavily during pregnancy. Sarah didn't drink at all during her pregnancy. Later on in Joshua Junior's life, he became an alcoholic, even though his father had stopped drinking altogether when Jr. was a toddler. Joshua Jr.'s molecular memory (genetic expression) now included a potential for alcoholism. Again, this is nurture affecting nature in the next generation.

Manesh's Story: music in my soul

Manesh grew up in Mumbai (Bombay), India, the eldest of nine children. His parents both worked in a clothing factory, where Bollywood classics were blaring on the stereo all day. When his parents came home in the evenings, they preferred conversation to music at the family table. The children's laughter and noisy chaos were sweet music to their parents' ears. Manesh was responsible for much of the child care while his parents were at work.

Manesh liked to play jazz music when cooking or cleaning, and there was only one local station on the radio that played it. For

Manesh, listening to jazz was a way to express the inexpressible, and this was his refuge, the way to help him take care of his responsibilities in a smooth, easy manner. Jazz seemed to make everything run better in his life.

When his parents came home, the music was turned off, in cooperation with their rules. Yet, night after night, for years, before he went to sleep, Manesh pressed the small transistor radio up against his head, and listened to jazz all night, softly. He dreamed of becoming a professional saxophone player, even though he had no instrument or music lessons. Nobody in his family was especially musical, and he had a horrid singing voice. (When the ritual prayers were sung, it was revealed that Manesh couldn't carry a tune.)

Manesh eventually married and had children of his own. All of his children were musical, from a very early age. When Manesh figured out that they had perfect pitch when singing, he put them in an after school program that included singing lessons, piano, and the harmonium. Manesh's youngest child, Ashvi, was smitten with jazz, like her father. She played jazz music on the stereo at home often. When Ashvi joined a band class in high school, she decided on the saxophone, even though she had never seen or played one before. Within weeks, she became a star soloist at the school. Ashvi is now a composer, and she performs in venues all over India, mixing classical Indian music with jazz from the 1940's and 1950's.

This is a perfect example of how our environment, when reinforced repeatedly, can influence the next generation's tendencies. This is epigenetics, the gene's expressing themselves to the best of their abilities even though there may be non-genetic factors influencing behavior or traits.

Personally, when I ponder on how epigenetics can be shown in practical terms, I think about the use of sunglasses and sunscreen. Did early man slather on sunscreen or don sunglasses in the Paleolithic era? Thousands of years ago these tools weren't in existence, no matter how light or dark the eyes and skin color were. If humans did get sunburned badly or squinted in the sunlight, they became accustomed to it, and were less affected by it. If humans did not get sunburned thousands of years ago, then the external process of us applying sunscreen and sunglasses habitually in the modern era is changing the sensitivity of our skin and eyes, and increases the need for those tools. I believe this repeated use in the past hundred years or so gave rise to the need for these tools, and if we don't use them we suffer physically. We have changed the genetics. We just aren't as tough as we used to be. (The environment has changed as well, with a thinner ozone level that makes the sun's rays more potent.)

> **A Wellness Wisdom:**
> **You have the power**
> **and the potential with**
> **every choice you make**
> **to affect the future in**
> **an impactful manner.**

Even our responses to stress affect our genes and our tendencies for physical illnesses. We humans are systemic beings, meaning every *system in our body works in relationship to other systems*. Nothing is in isolation. That said, our human existence in society is also systemic. Our survival and our ability to thrive are in relation to things outside of our bodies: our community systems, spiritual systems, electrical systems, financial systems, transportation systems, food systems, environmental systems, etc. That is why it is vitally important to be your *own* partner, by eating well, moving a lot, lifting heavy things, and practicing activities that reduce stress like yoga, meditation, or prayer.

We can use these things as a way to heal ourselves from the mental and physical struggles that plague us *now*, and by actively participating in positive, life affirming choices, we can positively affect generations to come at the genetic level.

"With great power comes great responsibility."
—Voltaire

We have to believe we possess that power first.

Can we reinvent ourselves? Science seems to think so, and that brings me great hope for those of us who want to get un-stuck in this life. Epigenetics provides hope for the generations to come too. Be your own partner. Own the belief and the hope that you will meet at the end of this book a *Happy, Healthy You.*

Chapter Twelve

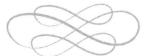

Depression vs. the Blues ~ Knowing the Difference Can Save Your Life or the Life of Someone You Love

What is depression? What are the blues? Why do some people experience life's challenges and have the blues for a short while, and why do others fall off the deep end and seem to really be down for a long time, or go back and forth into despair? We will answer these questions and many more in this chapter.

It may seem a little odd to be describing depression and the blues at this point in the book rather than in earlier chapters. I chose to describe these conditions here because the previous stories, exercises, therapies, and facts are indeed useful in treating the blues or depression. I didn't want the reader to get stuck on definitions and therapy terms. I prefer real humans and real stories. It will make more sense as one reads further, so read on!

What is depression?

Depression is a result of certain chemicals in the brain becoming imbalanced.[18] These chemicals, called neurotransmitters, are the regulators of emotions and behavior. If the neurotransmitters are imbalanced, then the emotions and behaviors of an individual will seem odd, sometimes severely odd, not only to others, but to themselves as well. This may go on for a prolonged period of time. The imbalances may be caused when certain life experiences occur. Examples of this may be a bad breakup, a death in the family, or other more traumatic ordeals like the ones described earlier in this book.

The brain is sensitive to external and internal environments. The nutrients we provide to our body affect the brain function as well. Illness and stress affect the normal functioning of the brain. Depression often runs in families too, which leads to a genetic predisposition to the illness. Hormonal changes and sleep disorders can cause depression. As explained in earlier chapters, our bodies are systemic in nature. All of our bodily systems can affect the brain, and the brain can affect all of our systems. It is not all bad news, however. We are not all destined for depression, even if it runs in the family (genetics, epigenetics). Being mindful, present, and being a partner with our bodies and our health care can make a huge difference in whether we suffer from the blues or from full blown depression after a traumatic event.

Symptoms of depression include:

- sad or irritable feelings most of the day

- loss of interest in most activities

- sleeping too much or too little

- weight loss or gain without trying

- thoughts of hopelessness and guilt

- thoughts of death and suicide

- inability to concentrate

- restlessness or sensation of living in slow motion

If one is depressed, it is hard to live with. It is hard on the depressed person's close circle of influence as well. The world seems gray. One has little to no motivation to do ANYTHING. Food has no taste. Socializing and the "old, happy" person have just disappeared. Physically and mentally one cannot enjoy participating in everyday life. When inside the depression, it is hard to realize it. One is just living it. Sometimes it is hard to imagine anything outside of the doom and gloom.

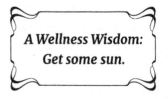

A Wellness Wisdom:
Get some sun.

It may take an outside friend or a close family member to recognize it and then take action to get help. If there is resistance (irritability), perhaps the first step may be to utilize the *Negative Thought Pot*. I describe this awareness tool in the introduction to this book. Do the exercise with the depressed person, so they know they are not alone, that everybody has things they want to release.

Another positive exercise I have shared with my coaching clients when they are depressed is walking outside in nature. See **Chapter 9** for more details on this technique. The friend or family member should walk with the depressed loved one instead of allowing him or her to be alone. Let's face it: he or she probably won't go for a nature walk alone anyway. The depressed person needs a loving push. It will do a world of good to connect with the environment in that way. Using the five senses when walking outside is so good for our central nervous system and the brain too. We also receive bursts of endorphins.[19]

The next step is to somehow get them to a helping professional, who can utilize talk therapy, medication therapy, somatic therapy, movement therapy, humor therapy, silent therapy, creative art therapy, etc. All these modalities are collaborative with the goal to make the depressed individual feel whole again. The goal is to rise and shine once more and to realize our superior selves.

Nutrition and Mood

Nutrition has so much of an effect on our mood that if we don't get enough of a certain mineral, vitamin, fat, or amino acid, we can rapidly fall into clinical depression.

If I ask you, "How will you feel, think, and behave if I withhold food from you for a day?" our conversation will be pretty predictable. You will be moody, angry, tired, fatigued, not able to concentrate on complicated tasks, etc. These are signs of depression, but it is only one day, so let's classify your reactions as the blues. Oh, you will probably be damn hungry too, and unable to sleep. (If you do fall asleep, you will probably dream of your next meal!)

The brain is fueled biochemically by the blood. The brain uses a lot of energy, therefore a lot of blood. The blood going into the brain affects the brain's performance, and therefore the body's performance. So the composition of the blood is very important. What we eat, drink, and absorb impacts the quality of the composition of the blood. This, in turn, impacts our awareness, our cognition, our ability to learn, our ability to be creative, and our ability to be loving, kind, and spiritual. It also impacts our ability to feel connected to others. Lack of real nutrient-dense foods for a prolonged period of time leads to a failure of these attributes and may cause depression.

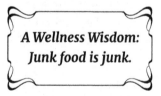

A Wellness Wisdom:
Junk food is junk.

Our blood is regenerated constantly, every day in fact. What we eat directly becomes what we think. This is why more modern societies with easy and cheap access to junk food have higher reports of anxiety and clinical depression. (JUNK FOOD=JUNK BLOOD=JUNK BRAIN) When we clean up our blood through our diet, we end up cleaning up our brains too. Everything works better.

Nowadays, most people's brains are suppressed. They are suppressed by toxins in our food and toxins in our environment. Food additives and preservatives are chemically altering our food and therefore our blood. Our personal care products and cleaning supplies are toxic as well.[20] We need to be aware of this in order to attend to our mental wellness. Those things we put in, on, and around ourselves are critical to our total health.

Foods and their Components Affecting Depression Symptoms

Here is a small sampling of some foods and their nutrients that directly affect our brain, our hormones, and our mental wellness. If someone is suffering from depression, some of these foods may enhance healing. Please seek out a health practitioner for further advice. Medication, psychotherapy, artistic therapies, and nutrition therapies often work very well together in rebalancing the chemical imbalances in the depressed person.

Foods that Support Brain Chemicals[21]

- **Dark, leafy greens** provide B vitamins, especially the B vitamin folate. Folate supports the feel-good chemical serotonin. Serotonin is manufactured in the brain and in the intestines. Serotonin is also considered a hormone. In fact, most of the neurotransmitters are acting as hormones throughout the brain and body. See **Chapter 14** for more detailed information on hormones. Serotonin provides a feeling of well being and happiness.

- **Meat, dairy, nuts, and dark chocolate** provide amino acids to the body and brain, especially tryptophan. Tryptophan breaks down further into serotonin and melatonin. Melatonin promotes calm and regulates our ability to fall asleep at the end of the day, when the sun sets. With the onset of artificial light sources, we have less melatonin being released by the brain, so we really need it from our food.

- **Chocolate** also increases the release of dopamine and endorphins. Dopamine is a pleasure generating hormone (neurotransmitter). Some say it is behind love, lust, motivation, and addiction. Endorphins are natural pain fighters and natural stress fighters. We may also feel high (euphoric) when endorphins are released in great quantities. Sex, meditation, and extreme athletic efforts may increase the levels of endorphins. Endorphins modulate our appetite and build immunity.

- **High protein sources like quality, grass fed meats, raw dairy and fats, wild fish, and wild seafood** protect against dopamine and norepinephrine deficiencies. When deficient in these two chemicals we feel extremely sluggish. Norepinephrine is the hormone responsible for maintaining normal blood pressure, heart rate, and sugar levels in the blood. One can see why deficiencies in these two hormones can find us tanking rather rapidly.

- **Fish and seafood** consumption assist in the absorption of Omega 3 fatty acids in the brain. The brain is comprised of over two thirds fat, so we really need healthy dietary fats to support its optimal function. In Japan, where more than 150 pounds of fish are consumed per person, per year, there is the lowest reported incidence of depression of any country in the world (2012).

- **Good mood fats like butter, chocolate, olive oil, avocado, coconut, fat from animals, and fat from nuts** also play an important part in brain health. Our ancestors had less adrenal stress and depression. They weren't eating the low fat, no fat diets, or processed, refined Franken-foods of our modern society. When we eat nonfat and low fat foods along with vegetables, we absorb less of the vegetables' vitamins, minerals, and phytochemicals. The opposite is also true. The more good fats eaten with vegetables, the higher bioavailability to the body. We need fat to absorb the fat soluble vitamins A, D, and E. Calcium cannot be absorbed by itself either. It needs fat.

This list is in no way comprehensive, but one can see here what an important contribution diet has on a person's entire well being. Multiple studies have been made in the past fifty years linking refined, processed foods to stress, obesity, and unfortunately, depression.

What About the Blues?

The blues, normal grieving, or sadness is a part of life. We will experience death, illness, disaster, embarrassment, and distress at different points in our lives. Even if we are lucky enough to be born with a silver spoon in our mouths, someone somewhere will disappoint us greatly. The times of deep sorrow allow us to appreciate life's blessings even more.

I think the difference between the blues and depression is that in the state of the blues the world seems empty. In the state of depression, *I* am empty.

The blues is a condition that is temporary. One can independently turn to others for comfort and consolation. Depression is pervasive and when one is inside of it, it seems to be endless. One often doesn't have the capacity to turn to others for help, either professional or otherwise. Many depressed people go undiagnosed or are embarrassed about seeking assistance.

Feeling down in the dumps doesn't interfere with regular, daily activities. One can feel melancholy and still get through the day, take care of his or her hygiene, go to work, cook, clean, take care of the family, etc. Feeling the blues for some time after a tragic life event is natural and normal. We know innately that we will bounce back. It is not a chemical imbalance like depression.

Suicide

If left undiagnosed or untreated, severe depression may lead
to suicide.

People who live in such internal pain and turmoil *do not want
to die*, as some would think. They just can't stand to live with the
hurt. Suicide attempters or successful suicide victims seem to have
run out of coping resources, even for those in therapies and on
medication. The people who carry out suicide see no other path to
healing from internal suffering.

Often times the one suffering in despair hides it for so long and
so well that even those closest to the depressed person have no clue
about what's going on in their heart, soul, mind, or brain...until it's
too late. Suicide is a very permanent solution to a non-permanent
problem. The family and friends never really have all the answers
when someone they love takes his or her own life. The suicide victim
takes all of the answers with him or her. Families are broken, family
systems are shattered, some never to be repaired.

It is my heart and soul wish that if anyone reading this is
suffering from deep despair, thoughts of suicide, or thoughts
of hurting oneself physically, seek immediate help from a crisis
center or call 9-1-1. I ask you to please reach out to a friend, family
member, religious leader, social worker, counselor, or medical
professional. Bare your soul and worries to them. You are not alone.
People care. They really do, way more than one would think.

My Story: post partum blues

When I had my first child, my son had problems latching on to my
breasts during nursing. This resulted in ninety minute bouts of
breastfeeding attempts, with milk flowing sometimes and sometimes
not, punctuated by frustrated cries. It was exhausting for both of us.

Daytime was tolerable for me in the beginning because I was high on birth hormones and the fact that I had a baby! It was the warm season where we lived (in San Francisco), and I made sure to get outside every day, walking up and down the steep hills in an effort to be positive, active, and get sunshine for vitamin D.

Nighttime was another story altogether. The ninety minute sessions resulted in me sleeping between one and a half to three hours nightly. After a few weeks I felt like I had left my body. I was totally wiped out. I was so sad and felt like a failure because I couldn't get this feeding thing down that looked so easy and natural in the videos and pictures. At mommy and me classes, other moms seemed to do it like pros the first time out of the gate. I began crying at the smallest things and could not bear to watch the news. My son would not sleep unless he was attached to my nipple, and I could not nap in the daytime. I never was a napper anyway. I felt like a zombie. The post partum hormones coupled with the lack of sleep brought me to the brink of my humanity. I reached out and had a teary, heart to heart phone call with a dear friend.

After the call, together, my friend and my husband packed the family up and headed to the doctor's office for help. We were educated on post partum depression and blues caused by hormonal changes, the lack of sleep causing other brain hormone imbalances, and the stress of new parenting causing the milk lactation to suffer. It is also called the baby blues. I learned most women feel a bit of the baby blues after giving birth.

We were given specific instructions on how to help the baby latch on to the breast better. The lactation specialist showed us exactly what to do. I taped a thin tube to my breasts to attach formula from a bottle attached to a baseball hat, so my boy would feel successful at what he was attempting to do (eat). It worked!

We were told to give me a strong Manhattan cocktail (my favorite at the time), and send me to bed for at least nine hours! Sleep was essential for my milk production and hormone balance. We were told which foods, supplements, and herbs were helpful for lactation and post partum stressors. We were informed that (luckily) most post partum depression and blues symptoms dissipate within a few weeks.

The environment and my relationships were extremely important to me at this time. Within a week, I felt a complete turnaround. My baby was eating more quantity in less time, I was sleeping better, and my mood lifted. I was on the road to recovery. If I had not recognized that sleeplessness, crying all the time, and not being able to watch the news was not normal, I do not know how far I would have traveled down the post partum depression path. I am wordlessly grateful for my phone call, my friend, and my husband's actions that day. They are a blessed example of what a tribe is capable of doing.

For a person suffering from depression, participating in activities that are pleasurable, or used to be pleasurable, releases memories *and* feel good hormones at the same time.[22] These are powerful mechanisms in healing. This wellness tool may not be independently available to a depressed person if she or he is all wrapped up in private thoughts. Encourage the sufferer to do things that you know are fun for him or her.

Remember that it is not any one's fault if one is in utter despair. He or she cannot just *snap out of it*. Depression is a mental illness.

There is a wealth of support services freely available on the internet. If it is an immediate crisis dial 9-1-1 or go to the nearest hospital.

Do not ignore your moods. Do not ignore your foods. They are intimately connected, as seen earlier. Do not ignore your health practitioner. Do not ignore your instincts. Educate yourself and surround yourself with people who love and support you. Get outside and play. Happiness is your birthright, but it is manufactured in the intestinal tract and in the brain.

"No man is an island, no man stands alone."
—Peter Schickele

The power of friends, family, mentors, and social circles is always vital in our lives, more so in a depressed person's life. All creatures are meant to live in clans of sorts, and even wandering ascetics come back to some group from time to time. Our species cannot survive with most people living in a group of one. Depression may cause a person to withdraw and seek isolation. The withdrawal may then further the depression. It bears repeating, the depressed person cannot just "snap out of it." As the saying goes, "It takes a village…"

"If you are depressed,
You are living in the past.
If you are anxious,
You are living in the future.
If you are at peace,
You are living in the present."
—Anonymous

Normal anxiety occurs with regular life stresses. We can self-regulate with action and self-restorative practices. These things take care of business, usually.

The symptoms of anxiety disorder may include:

- unexplained, constant worrying about the same things over and over again

- insomnia or restless sleep

- inability to eat or a decreased appetite

- increased sweat and rapid breathing

- panic attacks

If left unattended, the disturbed person may develop embarrassment or shame surrounding their symptoms and withdraw from social situations. If left untreated for a long period of time, anxiety disorder may lead to depression.

So many of the people in the previous stories shared in this book have gone down paths that would have led to serious behavioral symptoms had not somebody stepped in who really cared about them. The person who was sexually abused, the woman who suffered the death of her mother at a young age, the immigrant who walked hundreds of miles to safety through a war zone...they clung to something greater. They held true to their family, their friends, and their beliefs that something greater and bigger out there in the world was waiting to shine love and greatness upon them one day soon....You too have the capacity to be the higher spirit and human you were meant to be. Believe it, know it.

As the above quote so poetically phrased, we are all attempting to get to the present. That's the happy spot. Right here. Right now. I can't control what has already happened. It is dead. I can't control what is going to happen, despite my preparations (earthquake, hurricane, tragedy of war, anyone?). I can, however, be in this moment, and choose to be happy in it.

My thoughts are so damn powerful, and so are my choices. I choose to be peaceful, calm, and content, *now*. How about you? I invite you to join me in the *movement* of the *moment*. Cling to your support system, take baby steps, and ask for help. Move toward your *Happy, Healthy You.*

Chapter Thirteen

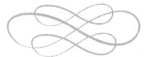

Loving Relationships as a Recovery Tool ~ Turn to Your Tribe of Support

Some people experience hardship and then just barely exist for the remainder of their lives. They are broken. Some do more than survive. They seem super human. They are the ones we look at in astonishment and wonder, and say, "See what they did after _____? How did they do that?

Wow. Just wow. They thrive. They super-survive. They take the reins of their lives and gallop forward, exceeding by far what they and anyone in their close circle expected after a trauma. Ordinary folks can make extraordinary strides in their lives.

I think it's a matter of making conscious, present-focused choices. We all have choices to make every moment. When we reach for positive choices, it is nature and nurture in harmony. It is a marriage of our past good experiences, and figuring out what our deepest desires are. It is very easy to become pessimistic after a tragedy. It is easy to feel hopeless. It is harder to choose growth and inner strength. Recognizing the path one is on right now is step one. If we have relationships that are loving and helpful, we can more easily move forward on that path.

"Be who you are and say what you feel, because those who mind don't matter, and those who matter don't mind."
—Anonymous

With loving supporters at our side, I believe we can acknowledge our deepest desires and take the first step onto the yellow brick road, moving forward toward the great and powerful Oz (you).

Chaz's Story

Chaz was plagued with severe mood swings from the early age of six. His parents and grandparents believed he would outgrow these mood swings. They thought that with lots of interventions, like play therapy, music therapy, and acting lessons, they could get a handle on the situation.

Both his parents and his grandparents on both sides of the family were artistic. They understood angst, exaltation, and everything in between. Rather than labeling the child, and predicting a negative, definitive outcome, the family loved him enough to work with him and obtain help from all of their loving relatives and teachers.

After six years of behavioral, emotional, occupational, and play therapies, the child rose above his earlier diagnoses. By age twelve, Chaz was known as a sensitive, brilliant actor in his school and community. He auditioned for every community theater project he could, and often got juicier roles than other children his age. The channeling of his mood swings into acting served him very well. The theatre was a safe place for Chaz to dig deep into his emotions without judgment from strangers as to whether his expression was appropriate. He could pull a variety of feelings out of a hat (so to speak) and compartmentalize them so that they didn't affect the rest of his day when he was not acting or in an improv class. Chaz didn't dwell in the dark parts of his existence. Chaz blossomed.

His family's choice was to actively seek out a solution with unconditional love as the basic foundation. Well, that was the key to his personal growth and healing. He was able to reorganize and redirect his mood swings into a balance. He became something greater than ordinary.

> *Remember that Chaz's family members were not necessarily victims themselves, suffering from great trauma or drama, or previously diagnosed with similar behavioral problems. They were still able to have great compassion and empathy for the child. We all can take the experiences of others, grow from their growth, use that growth, and change our own lives after hearing or witnessing their changes for the better. Sometimes being a fly on the wall ain't so bad after all.*

Adults spend a great deal of time with significant others outside of work. When we live with a partner, we learn how to observe their moods, emotions, and how to step in and show support. This reveals the strength of the relationship. When we are the other partner of a person suffering from emotional distress, we can help in many ways. Our first opportunity to help is by beginning with a conversation that is calm and loving.

We can say to our loved one, "Hey, I see you are not your usual self. Let's work on this together. I'm here for you. I am willing to do whatever it takes to bring you up to optimum life, energy, and happiness."

What a powerful, loving, empowering thing to do and say – to reach out. How can *we* (not point fingers) change up our lives, in order to feel better? Can you imagine how great life could be (to get this support from our lover)? This is amazing. This is saying, "I see you. I see how things could be, to make you the happiest that you can be. Let's roll up our sleeves *together* and make happiness happen."

"Tilt, don't wilt."
—Setarah, yoga instructor

This quote refers to the crescent moon pose where we reach up as tall as we can and create a beautiful arch towards all four sides of the room, while never collapsing the spine during the pose. For loving relationships as a recovery tool, the quote means that we can lean on our strong and significant others in our tribe without completely collapsing into their care, building enough inner strength to refrain from becoming codependent. Codependency is where a person leans on another or others for meeting all of his or her emotional needs, and for building his or her self-esteem from the bottom up. Codependency can also make the loved one who is helping feel like a super star. Be mindful.

It is never too late to change your life or your situation. If you have love as your ally, your free will's motor will be fired up, and you can get un-stuck, and be able to go after your goals, no matter what they are. This is the definition of well being. It is a wealth of health, happiness, and satisfaction. It is feeling connected to each other and to the bigger world out there.

Perhaps the best way to believe in the value of ourselves is to ask our closest pals to be our sounding board. You know who you trust. Go to them.

Statistics say that our relationships with others are the most influential source of life satisfaction.[23] This has been found across all ages and cultures worldwide. Great relationships make us more creative and provide us with challenges of every sort. If we work through these, we can work through stress and trauma too, with greater ease.

We must practice improving our relationships. We do this every day without even realizing it. We change our lives moment to moment, and we bring our loved ones along for the ride. It is very symbiotic and systemic, as discussed earlier.

An Invitation: relationship exercise

Think about who you love deeply and why. It does not have to be a romantic or sexual relationship. Now, write down who you love and three reasons why. Be honest. Define what sort of love it is, and what he or she gives to your overall well being. Do not judge them or yourself. It is all love.

Ask that person to do the same thing for you. Share your notes with each other. Smile. Breathe deeply. Accept that you are loved, despite your flaws. You are loved in many ways and for many reasons.

In a relationship that is good, we are drawn to the other person, and in the beginning, we can't get enough of them. We just suit up and show up, and we can't explain exactly why. It's that way for friendships and romantic relationships. It's that way for our gurus, our favorite leaders, our inspirations. If we channel our healing in that manner, we can move on from the past hurt. Make *healing*, itself, the new relationship.

Ivy's Story: the icing on the cake

Ivy is a friend I met at a library workshop a few years ago. The workshop theme was grain free/sugar free desserts. Afterwards, Ivy and I talked about desserts, especially our love of frosting and whipped cream. She shared with me her story of how she met her fiancé, Astor.

Two years earlier Ivy had met Astor at an art auction benefitting autistic children. The art was magnificent. The artists were the children themselves; their art showed the community of supporters how a label of autism does not define one's whole life.

Ivy was silently enjoying the art with a chocolate-dipped strawberry in hand, when a handsome man came up to her and silently handed her a cocktail napkin, gesturing to her chin. Ivy wiped the chocolate off of her chin, knowing that was what he meant by the gesture. They introduced themselves to each other and chatted the night away. Their first date followed a week later. Ivy told me that when Astor saw the chocolate on her chin and handed her a napkin, it was a compliment. He was taking care of her already. Other women might have seen it as a stranger pointing out their sloppiness or a flaw in their character.

Ivy went on to explain that on their first date, she said straight up to Astor, "I'm the cake. If you want to be the icing on my cake, you are welcome to be that. Remember, I'm the cake. And, you are the cake in your life. I can be the icing on your cake, but you are the cake. You are the main substance, your own core."

What a great way to start out a loving and stable relationship.

"Ideally, couples need three lives; one for him, one for her, and for them together."
—Jaqueline Bisset, actor

My mentor, Colin F. Watson, says we must suit up and show up in order to move on (I say, every damn day.). I add that *sometimes* we must reverse this: *we must move on in order to show up in our own healing.* What this means is that we need to figure out what has just happened to us that wasn't so pleasant at *another* time. Keep moving forward away from nasty-land and towards loving-land. The answers, analysis, awareness, and realizations will come to fruition in their own time, if we devote energy to them later. But, get yourself to a safe place, now. Then, when we least expect it, the *aha* moment will show up. And then we will make sense of it all. Keep your little notebook handy.

After all, you are bringing your whole self with you. Everywhere you go, there you are. Perhaps by *not* sprinting away from the confusions and misunderstandings that this life gives us freely, but steadily and calmly moving in the direction we want our lives to go, we will *want* to face our true selves. Hello, *you.*

An Invitation: getting to know you

Pretend you have never met yourself. You are meeting yourself for the first time, like in a class or in the grocery store produce section.

Write down your three strongest pet peeves and why. Explain this so the person who has never met you before will get to know you better.

Write down three things someone would be surprised to know about you. What do these things say about you? These three things can help us reacquaint ourselves with who we are at our core, our personal values, and the personal history that shapes us, even though we are changing and growing (hopefully for the better) moment to moment.

There are powerful forces within us that resist change, even though we know it would be beneficial for us. We do things over and over again whether or not we are gaining energy and knowledge from those activities just because we have always done them that way. Comfort, convenience, and the familiar routines feel safe, but may not always serve your higher purpose. This book is here to show you that this reasoning is not good enough for you, now that you do not want to remain paralyzed in your life. What do we need to do? We need to confront our fears and create new rules with our loved ones at our back. People say that they have your back all the time. Take them at their word. They are waiting for a *Happy, Healthy You.*

Chapter Fourteen

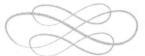

Hormones and Wellness ~ The Rulers of Our Bodies We Didn't Even Know About

We have all heard of hormones. What are they exactly? How do they help or impair our goal of living life happily and recovering from stress, family drama, or trauma? How can they play a role in our gusto in going after our life goals?

Hormones are messengers that carry particular messages from one part of the body to another; they travel mostly through the bloodstream, and sometimes through the nervous system. Most hormones are secreted by glands, and this glandular system is called the endocrine system. Hormones are made of proteins, amino acids, and cholesterol (yes, we need cholesterol...the body wouldn't produce it if we didn't need it).

Hormones rule every part of our bodies. They control our growth, weight, metabolism, fertility, and water levels. They begin puberty and end the fertility stage when appropriate. They tell us when to be attracted to someone, when to fall in love, when to have sex, and when to run like hell! Hormones control our emotions and moods.[24]

As discussed earlier in this book, all of the systems within our bodies are related to other systems. We are not doing one thing in isolation. So, if I tell you to just stop doing everything, and to focus on your breath, you cannot do just that one thing. Your respiratory system will keep you inhaling and exhaling so you will have oxygen passing through your body. Your cardiovascular system will still pump your heart and move fresh, oxygenated blood throughout the body. Your skin will still perspire on its own if it is warm outside and you are moving briskly.

The endocrine system sends hormones, its messengers, through the blood to the part of the body that is ready to receive the message from the brain. The brain receives all of the information we experience and sense. Then, the brain decides what to do with the information. The brain is the master gland, the master planner behind all the other glands. Then, the pituitary gland in the brain sends out the task at hand, once the decision is made.

Hormones can be created in fat cells, tissue cells, muscles, in the liver, and even in the skin. Scientists are discovering more and more hormones each year. There were only a few dozen hormones identified not many years ago, and now there are more than a hundred identified hormones.

Our activities outside the body have a direct effect on the hormones inside the body. Things like stress, sleep, exercise, eating, sex, studying, etc. have a huge impact on hormonal function, balance, and imbalance.

The Basics of the Endocrine System[25]

The better known, classic glands and organs that tell the hormones to carry particular messages are:

- **the brain, the master planner**

- **the pituitary gland, at the base of the hypothalamus**

- the thyroid gland

- the parathyroid gland

- the pancreas

- the adrenal glands

- the intestines

- the placenta

- the testes or ovaries (gender specific)

These body parts each produce particular hormones in order to make the body function in the way it was designed.

The **pituitary gland** has many tasks. It secretes prolactin, which tells the mammary glands to produce milk for breastfeeding. It also releases a hormone which tells the adrenal glands to produce cortisol, the fight or flight hormone. The pituitary releases growth hormones for our bodies to grow into adulthood, and regulates body composition and metabolism. The hypothalamus works in conjunction with the pituitary gland. This gland also produces a thyroid stimulating hormone, which stimulates the thyroid and tells the thyroid to secrete its own hormones.

The **thyroid gland** secretes thyroxin (T4) and triiodothyronine (T3). The thyroid needs iodine in order to make these hormones. We usually get iodine from food, but if needed, the thyroid can pull it from the body's stores. These hormones control metabolism and energy balance. Metabolism is how fast or slow our body burns fuel (food) for our daily activities.

The **parathyroid gland** releases parathyroid hormone: this controls the calcium levels in our body. If we need calcium and we cannot absorb it from our food, our parathyroid will pull calcium from our bones to do the work it needs to do.

The **pancreas** secretes insulin and glucagon hormones. When sugar levels in the bloodstream are high, the pancreas secretes insulin to balance out the sugar high. When sugar levels in the bloodstream are low, the pancreas releases glucagon to bring up sugar levels and create balance of energy. These two hormones reach every part of the body.

The **adrenal glands** secrete androgens and the stress hormone cortisol. When we are in great fear or danger, these hormones allow us to survive, think fast on our feet, and produce an action that will yield our best survival result (hopefully). The adrenal glands also produce adrenaline, epinephrine, and dopamine, as well as rushes of energy hormones, and pleasure hormones. There are many more hormones the adrenals make, but we are just covering the basics here.

The **intestines** secrete a hormone called cholecystokinin, which helps with digestion, pancreatic enzymes and bile production. The intestines also produce secretin, which helps with digestion and absorption of nutrients, and neutralizes acid.

The **placenta** is a temporary endocrine gland. During pregnancy, this gland makes hormones that are important for the growth and development of the fetus, as well as making hormones to protect the mother during pregnancy. The hormone oestrogen and progesterone are made here. Oestrogen stimulates the growth of the uterus to make space for the growing fetus, as well as stimulating the mammary glands. Progesterone makes the lining of the uterus a healthy place for the baby to grow. Human chorionic gonadotrophin (HCG) is made in the placenta too, and if the mother is malnourished during pregnancy, the HCG hormone will mobilize the mother's abnormal fat stores to be utilized as food for the fetus.

The **sex glands**, which are the **testes** in men, and the **ovaries** in women, secrete hormones vital for our sex drive (libido), and for the overall development of our sex and fertility organs. In men, the testes secrete testosterone, which is responsible for the development of maleness in boys; the change in hair, body odor, and voice as they grow through puberty. Testosterone aids in the maintenance of muscle strength and bone density throughout life. In women, the ovaries are the counterpart to the testes. The ovaries release two main hormones, estrogen and progesterone. Estrogen is what contributes to femaleness, in body changes such as hair, body odor, breast growth, and so forth during puberty. Progesterone prepares the uterus for menstruation each month, and protects fertility.

This list seems endless, and we have just gotten started. How are we to make sense of all of these hormones? How can they affect our ability to be well, mentally and spiritually too? How can we heal from our deep pain and suffering if we are perhaps out of balance hormonally?

Well, luckily for us, our body is remarkable in that it seeks balance all of the time, in all areas, and in all systems. This balance is called homeostasis. I want us to get a basic understanding of hormones so that we may attend to taking care of them.

The easiest and most functional way of caring for our hormones and the work they do is to eat well and move often. Again, it all keeps coming back to nutrient dense, real foods, controlling our stress levels through focused relaxation and movement, and finally, getting outside and spending time in nature. If we find out through symptoms and testing that our hormones are imbalanced, we can attend to the healing of the hormone imbalance.

Sometimes the mental and physical issues can be healed through good nutrition.[26] Supplements may help as well. In many cases, these conditions and imbalances can be reversed by paying close attention to the symptoms, as well as working with a holistic, functional endocrinologist. As shared earlier, there are common threads of healing present in restorative practices such as yoga, which has been found to improve the endocrine system.

When we eat well, live well, and laugh often, our general mood (and life) is happier and in balance. Then we can focus on the real life challenges we want to attend to with a strong constitution. On the other hand, in this modern world of moving at the speed of thought, multimedia coming at us every second with texts, tweets, and messages...well, the daily tasks seem to be complicated, as do our relationships. We have a daunting task to accomplish this delicate balance.

There's an old cliché heard around the globe, "Happy wife, happy life!" To this I add, "Happy hormones, happy wife!" Our moods are regulated by this wonderful symphony orchestra of the endocrine system, led by the brain as the master conductor. Men's moods are affected by hormones as well, but for some reason, we speak about women more often in the discussion of hormones.

Bianca's Story: I can't even get Thursday right

Bianca had a wonderful time at dinner with her friends last night after work. She had a healthy seafood dinner with a glass or two of wine, followed by dessert and coffee. She had coffee around 8 p.m. When Bianca went to bed at 10:30 p.m, she couldn't fall asleep. It may have been the coffee or the alcohol or the sugar, but whatever the culprit, she couldn't sleep. Not enough melatonin (sleep hormone) was being released by her pituitary gland; finally she passed out around 4 a.m.

Her alarm clock, however, was set for 7:15 a.m., her regular wakeup time. Cortisol is responsible for waking us up to use the restroom in the middle of the night, and for awakening us in the morning. She didn't get enough sleep the night before, resulting in less cortisol (if any) being released to wake Bianca up. Then she felt sluggish and grumpy all day. She had an extra cup or two of coffee to get her through to 5 p.m.

Then, when the false energy source of caffeine crashed, she had a mood swing into the sad, tired zone. No worries! Bianca grabbed another cup of coffee and a cinnamon roll on her way out of the office. The coffee with cream and sugar, cinnamon roll with extra icing, and the handful of chocolate chips turned into sugar in her bloodstream. Then her body released a surge of insulin to deal with that sugar.

Traffic is heavy, and Bianca is THIS close to getting side swiped by someone changing lanes on the freeway. Adding to her stress was the daycare provider's rule: children must be picked up by 6 p.m., or face penalties of a dollar a minute overtime. Her cortisol has skyrocketed and her bloodstream is a mess. The ancestral human fight-or-flight response has been aroused because she is stuck in traffic. Bianca can do neither. Between the cortisol and the insulin, the extra sugar will be turned into fat. Her body biologically does not know when she will be in a safe place of calm again.

Our body holds only a teaspoon of glucose in the entire bloodstream at any one time. If Bianca isn't using the energy provided by the sweets and coffee right away, the hormones will assist by turning the excess glucose into stored fat. Now, how will that make her feel?

Is this good for her self-esteem? No. Is this good for her stress? No. Is this good for her bitchy, crabby demeanor when she picks up her child at 6:29 p.m.? No. Does this make her calm and patient when she arrives home to spend quality time with her significant other? No. So, how in the *Sam Hell* is she supposed to deal with her past neglect, abuse, trauma, or drama, when she can't even get Thursday right?

Our natural hormone secretions and their delicate balances may be interrupted by poor food choices, cosmetics, lotions, plastics, household chemicals, and environmental pollution. We are exposed to 84,000 man-made chemicals on a daily basis (on average), yet only 200 of these chemicals have been tested by the Environmental Protection Agency. The most common endocrine disruptor is the hormone estrogen, which is found in almost everything, from soy to beer, from sunscreen to soil.[27] Most of us have too much estrogen in our bodies at any one time.

We *can* participate in regulating our external levels of hormonal intake by reading the labels on what we use in and around our bodies. We *can* regulate our sleep/wake cycles more efficiently to assist in the balance of those hormones. Read the ingredients of the food you bring home, and read the ingredients of the lotions and potions used by your family. Seek out the assistance of a functional endocrinologist, a doctor who specializes in the optimal levels of the endocrine system, rather than just the diseases of the endocrine system.

Sometimes, despite the great care and attention we place upon our health and vitality, we may still have hormonal imbalances. I recently found out that I have hypothyroidism, a lack of the thyroid gland doing its job. I eat extremely clean and green. I practice yoga and meditation almost daily. I spend lots of time outdoors in nature. I practice stress reduction techniques. I lift heavy things. I sleep nine to ten hours a night. I pay attention to the lotions and potions I use in my body and around my home. I read detailed ingredient lists on almost every product.

My doctor said most likely my condition was hereditary. My mom had thyroid dysfunction and thyroid cancer, and other members of my family have other hormonal dysfunctions.

Perhaps I was keenly aware of my symptoms and knew exactly what blood tests to ask for because of my clean eating and living routine. Maybe I wouldn't have even noticed the symptoms if I had been on a bagel, pizza, and cake (with sugar-free cola) eating protocol.

Now, I am actively involved as a partner with my practitioner in getting my endocrine system back to optimal function. I am not beating myself up with the information, or trying to play the blame game and figure out what I could have done differently in the years before I cleaned up my act. The information is just that: information. And, it is empowering me *now* to take control of my situation in a calm and methodical manner; body, soul and mind.

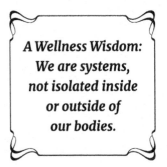

A Wellness Wisdom:
We are systems,
not isolated inside
or outside of
our bodies.

The list of glands and hormones described here is by no means exhaustive. This is just the tip of the iceberg. I want you, the reader, to have a basic understanding of our hormones and how they work, in harmony or in disharmony. I want this to be accessible to the general public, so that we may make smarter choices when dealing with unnecessary hormones found in processed factory foods (including animal products), chemicals, air and water pollutants, cosmetics, and lotions. I want you to see the correlation between our hormonal balances and lifestyle choices like sleep, rest, and activity.

My dear readers, we have a huge task to attend to: to care for our biology in order to be able to attempt to care for our psychology.

When Benjamin Franklin said, "An ounce of prevention is worth a pound of cure," he was referring to preventing fires in Philadelphia, which was at that time an unsafe city. In our present day world, we too, need to be educated about environmental dangers, and organize ourselves to the point that if a personal crisis comes up, we may respond rather than remain paralyzed. Our world runs faster and faster than ever, and is more demanding too. Let us stand tall and walk calmly and confidently together toward a *Happy, Healthy You.*

Chapter Fifteen

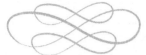

Somatic Therapy ~ Body Talk

Traditional psychotherapy is a talk based therapy. When we experience traumatic crises and choose traditional therapy to work through it all, we spend time talking with another person, talking through the feelings and emotions related to and from the event. Our state of turmoil and feelings of paralysis in our lives are acknowledged in a very heady way. We live in our head most of the time anyway.

Usually the mind doctor and the body doctor are two separate visits. When we have an ache or pain, a broken bone or cancer, we go to a physical specialist. When we have stress or deep hurt in our heart, we go to a mental specialist.

As described earlier in this book, our mind affects our nervous system, our endocrine system, and all of the chemicals released throughout the body. All of our systems are intertwined in their actions and reactions. We are biologically and physically affected by external and internal circumstances. It makes sense then that our entire well-being would benefit from attention in a combined, integrative manner. The body/mind connection in healing may be called "somatic." Somatic experience is when we notice the bodily reactions *first* (surrounding a memory or feeling). This type of coaching has been practiced for about 45 years.[28]

Somatic psychotherapy is a form of body oriented therapy. Somatic therapy works through challenges by acknowledging that the physical body holds clues and answers to the problems and stressors. We attend to our struggles through discussion, as well as through shifting the attention towards tensions and movements and following with relaxation exercises. This, in turn, helps the mind heal from the past crises. Somatic therapy is holistic in nature, and considers the mind, body, and spiritual approaches to healing.

Many of the previous exercises in this book may be considered to be somatic exercises.

When I think of the meditative, trance-like, nirvana state of spinning in a circle, over and over again, like whirling dervishes, I see this as a form of somatic therapy. The spiritual aspect of whirling, along with remembering a problem or a prayer for something we want to resolve, can be the physical release we need. We can unfreeze the energy. We can feel freedom from the pain and hurt through the spinning. If we add music or whirl outdoors, we may add another level of healing to our immediate environment. Our bodies physiologically react to trauma, so we can physically take action in order to heal from trauma.

⤳⧓⤳

Greta's Story: seen and not heard

Greta seemed skittish and nervous speaking in public during elementary school. As a child, her parents didn't put much value in Greta's contributions to family discussions at the dinner table. They were pretty old school in their approach to child rearing: *children should be seen and not heard.*

This was all Greta knew growing up, so that particular dogma was instilled in her. It was also her survival tool; subscribe to these rules and beliefs in order to not get into trouble with her elders. She was a well behaved child and did what she was told.

Now, as an adult in her mid-thirties, Greta was a great team player at work where she was an administrative assistant. Everybody knew that Greta did much of the work for her boss, and that her boss would not survive the week without Greta's savvy. For seven years, Greta was overlooked for a promotion. She received pay raises, but never a new title or accolades. Greta was frustrated and frequently getting migraines. The frustration led to chronic lower back pain, acid reflux, and a host of other minor symptoms related to the stress at work.

When I met Greta, at a library workshop on getting ahead in business, we clicked. We decided to work together on her frustrations. We began by meeting at Lake Merced in San Francisco. We had a plan to race-walk and talk. Before we began walking around the lake, I asked her to lie on her back on top of the picnic table, near where the seagulls hung out. I told her to close her eyes and inhale deeply through her nose.

I then asked Greta what she really wanted out of our time together. She told me that she wanted to have the courage to ask for a promotion at the company meeting coming up. She wanted to state her desire and qualifications in front of about forty people at the meeting, and she was terrified.

We practiced the scenario with Greta lying on the table in the warm sun, in a non-threatening, natural, uplifting environment. As Greta practiced her speech, I noticed her breathing becoming rapid and shallow, her face beginning to get red with embarrassment or shame, and her body beginning to fidget. I asked Greta to scan her body to notice these physical things happening and to just be aware of them.

Then I asked her to focus on slowing down her breath and to only breathe in and out of her nose to the count of six. I told her to place her hands on any areas of tension and feel the warmth and comfort of her hands there. Together we worked through relaxing the tense parts of her body. We acknowledged that the stress came from her past experiences as a child, but that the child is not who she is right now. That dogma doesn't serve her now. We adjusted the physical as a way of releasing the mental bonds that kept her stuck.

Greta's attention to her body first changed her internal dialogue and beliefs about what she deserved, and about what she could or could not accomplish. She moved and behaved little by little in a more confident and assertive way, not like the meek little girl she once was, living under the rules and expectations of long ago. After about eight weeks of practicing and visualizing with me once a week, walking around the beautiful lake, and gaining the benefits of being out in nature, Greta became a different woman. Her aches and pains subsided, she asked for and received the promotion she so deserved, and a new sense of freedom emerged.

⚬⚬⚬

Greta's story is an example of somatic therapy. We focused on the body to assist in tackling the internal strife. For some reason, we humans say, "Seeing is believing." We always ask for proof. At the same time we ask for belief in the unseen...like *love*, *God*, *breath*, *bliss*, or *enlightenment*. This type of therapy allows for proof to be given to us through the body shift, before the mind shifts.

Greta felt that what she accomplished was a miracle, considering how long she had held her "less than" beliefs. What we call miracles in healing are actually our belief systems being shifted into a new internal language. Placing the *attention* on the *intention* went beyond biology and psychology as two separate things. Was it a *miracle*, or just a series of realized potentials that we haven't quite labeled yet in science?

"If I'm too strong for some people, that's their problem." —Glenda Jackson, actor

Negativity and cynicism run rampant in our world. Think about the possibilities if we were to suspend the old dogmas and physically change our movements and reactions surrounding the negative thoughts that pop up. Somatic therapy allows us to regain our lives and reset our resilience. It integrates the body world, and affects the mind world.

Dance therapy, yoga therapy, laughter therapy, meditation, whirling, running, and shamanic therapy are all ways to integrate somatic therapy for total health. When we feel interior wholeness after working on the exterior levels, we can have a different kind of life than we ever thought possible. There is a whole world of sensory experiences out there that will acknowledge our hurt in a safe manner and release or free our pain, if we allow ourselves to do the work and then feel the feelings. Suppressing feelings serves no one, and suppressing feelings may destroy ourselves as well as those we love.

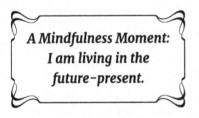

*A Mindfulness Moment:
I am living in the
future–present.*

Our external bodies are our artistic expressions of our internal life. How we dance, how we move through sports, how we dress, what makeup we wear, our jewelry choices, and our hair style and hair color choices are all part of our external expression of our internal life (piercings and tattoos, too). Sometimes we just have to trick ourselves, and project to the outside world who we desire to be perceived as, through these expressions, before it actually occurs. We *can* live in the future-present and *fake it 'til we make it!*

My cousin Annie, a salon owner, always says that hairdressers, nail artists, and aestheticians are also armchair psychologists. The focused attention and healing power of touch for an hour or more is a recovery tool as well. I agree.

Before I drive to work for my serving job, if I get a feeling in the pit of my stomach that the work day is going to be crappy, I physically do something about my attitude and my instinct. I put on glittery eye shadow, and add a little extra to my temples. I decided long ago (divine inspiration) that if I wear glitter, I can't possibly have a bad day. So, rather than fall down the rabbit hole of doom and gloom, I somatically have reactions to the glittery choice I make. Then I have internal changes based upon that. It works on my mindset every time. When I catch my reflection in the mirror at work, I think to myself, "I'm sparkling and glittery. I cannot have a bad day. I'm having a brilliant day, literally and figuratively." Then, I do. My body language changes to match the brilliance. I stand tall and proud. I smile more. Physically I shift, and then my expectations change. Remember, dear reader, expectations can help *or* hinder us.

Me and Betty Lee: great expectations

When I was going into the gym parking garage a few months ago, the lot was packed. There was a line of cars waiting for the sweaty gym rats to leave so the waiting gym members could take their parking spaces. I was crunched for time so I decided to go around all of the waiting cars and look for parking on the street. As I went out of line to exit, one car honked and honked at me! The driver rolled down the window and started yelling, "Hey! I was waiting for that spot!"

I rolled down my window and gave the woman the biggest smile I could muster and replied, "I would never take your spot! I'm going to exit the garage and park on the street!"

She said nothing in return, but her face turned red as she pulled into her coveted spot. We met again ten minutes later in the ladies' locker room. I walked directly up to her and introduced myself. She stammered out an apology and explained that she fully expected me to bogart her in the parking garage. Then she told me her name: Betty Lee. I shared with her that I was not the kind of human being to steal parking spaces, and I didn't want to be viewed in that way, ever. When I did not act as she originally expected, her body physically reacted with redness and silence. That was clearly a somatic experience for her. When I introduced myself in a calm, non-confrontational manner, her mind changed, her body language changed, and we became friends.

Ah, the lessons of expectations. Now, months later, every time I see Betty Lee at the gym, we stop and take the time to chat about our kids, husbands, travel, fitness, etc. The bond we created was built upon misinterpreted expectations!

My Story: feeling fear, failure, and real vulnerability in front of my children

I was born with a spinal condition called spondylolisthesis. It is where one bone is protruding off track, and in my case is moved forward on the spinal cord in front of it a little to the left. I had no clue I even had the disorder until third grade when I chose to play trumpet. The instrument was heavy and to carry the case home and to school daily along with my back pack created back aches. I had to give up the trumpet. My dreams of being a guest on the *Tony Orlando and Dawn* show were crushed.

Later on in ninth grade my left leg went entirely numb, caused by the bone pressing on the nerve which controlled the leg's function. I dragged my leg along behind me. The doctors suggested I lie flat on my back for a month as a non-invasive attempt to relax the bone off of the spinal cord and nerve. It worked. I was thrilled. I could walk normally again. The docs told me that in order to keep a strong spine I had to strengthen my core, my abdomen. The fitness world came into my life at age thirteen, and hasn't left since.

Just last year, after a yoga class I could not get up from the floor. I literally was in too much pain. I saw stars, and could not breathe. I received help to my car from the staff, and after a few days back and forth to the emergency room, it was revealed that the padding in between the spondylolisthesis bone had slipped on both sides, which was now causing slipped disc issues as well.

My sweet and dedicated son, Golden, who was fifteen years old at the time, would not leave my side when I went to the doc or emergency room. I told him to take a ride share service or a taxi and go have fun with his friends because my husband was out of town, but he was determined to be my support. One time we were in the hospital emergency room over five hours trying to come up with a plan of relief that didn't make me faint. I had fainted from some pain pills and muscle relaxers, and others made me itchy or caused insomnia. This ordeal lasted a month.

I was beginning to have the downward spiral of negative thoughts in my head, even though I am the positive energy gal. I was so afraid. The pain was so intense that it hurt to inhale. I could not walk. I could not drive. I could not turn over in bed without help. It hurt to yawn, but I desperately needed to yawn. I could not work as a server for a month. I had to use the *Negative Thought Pot* multiple times. I kept thinking, "I eat well, I do yoga, I hike, I sleep well, I even have my hormones under control. Why me, Lord? Why me?" I cried. I slept. I stayed in bed for nine days, except for appointments with doctors or massage therapists. I tried every aromatherapy, affirmation, meditation, medication, and motivation technique I could muster up.

I was a failure. I felt like I was a let down to my family and my tribe of followers. I thought I was going to live out my days in a bed or wheelchair like my mother, who was 89 years old. Then, one day after I fainted at the cell phone store at the mall (pain medicine too strong, not enough food), my son walked over from school to meet me there because I could not drive after fainting. Golden calmly took my hand and pressed on the padded muscle near the thumb. He said I needed to eat rice and vegetables and fish. He put his arm around me and gingerly took me to the healthy Korean place at the food court.

> **A Wellness Wisdom:**
> **There are times when**
> **we have to move our**
> **ego out of the way.**

I was keenly aware that I probably wasn't the strong mama bear figure he knew so well. I was learning that being vulnerable with your children is a new layer of trust, another level of the relationship. The fragility I felt as my immediate world crumbled was dispersing with the comfort of his healing somatic touch. Golden's hand was holding mine, and his gangly arm was draped around me in a protective fashion, for the first time ever. My body settled into the seat as I slowly tucked into my food. I held my right palm over my stomach area attempting to breathe in calm and exhale worry. Then after I was done eating, I took my left palm and placed it on my back at the source of the pain and talked to my back as if to an old friend I was breaking up with.

Eventually, the somatic touch therapy, along with cannabinoids oil, and epidural shots to the spine helped tremendously. I had to utilize many tools at once from the wellness toolkit, along with western medicine. The point was, and is, to get better, to get unstuck, to heal, to thrive, to become a *Happy, Healthy Me*.

Biocognitive Therapy: cultural leaning

When we take into consideration one's cultural background, and add that foundation to somatic therapy, healing may be brought up to another level of understanding. It is called Biocognitive Therapy. The belief systems and patterns that keep us stuck may have been planted by our culture generations before our birth. We do not have to subscribe to that forever though.

Dr. Mario Martinez coined the term biocognition. This means our minds and bodies work together in the filter of our culture.[29] The immune system and the belief system affect each other inside of a cultural community. The cultural context determines how our biology works out. Does the culture support or degrade our health?

Dr. Martinez explains biocognition with examples of women in menopause in two cultures: Peru and Japan. In Peru, the words for menopause and hot flashes during menopause mean "shame." It has been clinically found that the immune system in these women reacts by becoming inflammatory during this time of their lives. All of the inflammatory conditions like arthritis, headaches, joint aches, muscle pain, etc. increase during this time. Contrary to that, in Japan, the word for menopause means "second spring." Women are heeded as more wise during this time of their lives and as a resource for knowledge in the community. It has been found that the women's hot flashes are less severe, and their bodies are non-inflammatory, even during the hot flashes. The biology follows the cultural belief system. Women in Peru have a tougher time physically and mentally while going through the change of life than their Japanese counterparts.[30]

Think about these archetypal phrases in the USA: "I can't stomach that. I can't stand that person. You make me sick." These idioms are peculiar to our culture. When we get around a person who is the very embodiment of those statements, the body reacts in the way that we believe. When we affirm those beliefs repeatedly, we see our appetite diminishing and our stomach turning sour, and we feel tired and need to sit down. The body expresses what we said or thought and what we believe to be true, in these culturally shaped clichés. This is another example of biocognition.

These are practical terms and tools to know for our own lives. We can take the parts of our culture that do not serve us and mentally set them aside. We may create empowering thoughts instead, which, *when repeated,* change brain patterns, and in time, change the biology. We can manifest better outcomes in our bodies and in our minds. With practice, we can recover and heal from trauma and drama. Then we can create wellness and fulfillment.

I invite you to use your body to access your mind, becoming a *Happy, Healthy You.*

Chapter Sixteen

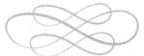

Positive Psychology ~ Say Yes to Yourself

What is Positive Psychology? How can it help us in our daily lives?

There are many ways of healing from every day stresses, life's tougher challenges, and even severe trauma. In earlier chapters we learned about talk therapies, healing through art, writing, role play, physical movement, music, silence, humor, and more.

Traditional psychology and psychotherapy focus on what is wrong in a person's life. They look at problems and seek to learn the source of the problems as a way to begin the point of the healing. Positive Psychology is a study and technique which focuses instead on a person's strengths rather than a person's weaknesses.[31] In a therapy session, a therapist and patient concentrate on what makes life worth living and what values bring deep meaning to the patient's life, despite the crappy things that brought them there in the first place. Rather than look at what is going wrong in one's life and the source of the beginning point of that, the therapist may ask how the patient reacted that was positive in any way to the negative experience, even if it was small or remotely linked. Then together, the patient and therapist build upon that for healing.

We inherently want to be happy. We have the right to be happy. We are born happy (most of us). It is our natural state. If we can remember the life experiences which make us positive and happy, the memories can trigger positive emotions in the present and influence our thinking and behavior now and in the future. If we can sit in the seat of well being for a few minutes a day, little-by-little we can let go of the horrible situations, and the subsequent feelings and emotions which do not serve us. Then we may build upon our strengths, passions, and positive experiences which do serve us. Positive Psychology is a science.[32] It is not just a way to...*think happy thoughts and things will get better.*

How do we know what our strengths are? Our strengths are those things we do that never make it to our "to do" list. We passionately and naturally flow with those tasks because they are part of the fabric of who we are. Our strengths never feel like work. For me, those strengths would include nurturing others, a love of learning, writing, teaching, and anything fitness related. Our strengths may lead to a steady state hum of happiness buzzing just under the surface of our existence, residing there while the rest of our busy lives reside up top.

An Invitation: strengths

Make a list of things you do that are your easy, joyful passions, and those things that never make your "to do" list. These are your strengths. Your strengths are your foundation. When you feel low from a bout of illness or a crappy day, it is nice to know one has something like this list to lean on. When the $#!+ hits the fan, revisit the list, nod, and say, "Yes. I can. I am awesome and strong." It is okay to be okay. We do not need validation from others to be okay, to be whole.

Strengths lead to positive emotions like joy, bliss, humor, awe, hope, contentment, pride, confidence, gratitude, a better attitude, and peace. Strengths and their resulting positive emotions have been studied throughout the years. Our strengths can prevent stress and depression across many socioeconomic areas.[33] Positive Psychology is sometimes also called Happiness Psychology.

Happiness is not selfish at all. It is quite healthy. In fact, positive emotions lower the stress hormones, reduce the heart rate, boost the immune system, and reduce perceived and actual pain levels. Another added bonus of positive emotions is that they are quite contagious! If someone else is feeling low, the positive person usually rubs off on them more than the other way around.

Positive Psychology doesn't necessarily have to occur in a therapist's office. Whether one is suffering or not, the techniques here can keep one from ever falling into heavy anxiety or depression in the first place. It is preventive in nature. There are many resources available to the general public for gaining excellent results from Positive Psychology. Every bookstore I visit has a section on self-help, happiness theories, and activity based psychology to try for oneself. In our modern society, there's even an app for that! I like the app called Happify. Happify has science-based activities and games to elevate happiness using Positive Psychology.

Everyone knows a "Negative Nancy." We all have been around pessimistic people at work, at school, and at social events. There are some who always complain about every little thing, even during a beautiful moment, and then it ruins the essence of the moment and the intention, and everyone in the room is left a bit deflated. It's not fun, it doesn't feel good, and it is contagious. It can snowball out of control. Walk away as fast as you can. That is my advice.

On the other hand, we all know people who are always upbeat and seem to have a skip in their step. They have a ready, wide smile, no matter what the weather. When asked how they are doing, their answer is usually, "Fabulous!" Surround yourself with these sorts of people, especially if attempting to inject Positive Psychology into your daily life. Positive Psychology *can* be learned. It is a conscious, mindful effort that takes practice. We will live with more resilience and share more of that resilience with others with daily repetition of positive actions. I see it in my coaching practice, and I practice it in my own life.

Acceptance: Bad Things Sometimes Happen

If we practice Positive Psychology, with repetition, we will experience so many positive emotions and strengths, thus boosting our sense of normalcy. We may feel super human. A general hum of happiness ensues. When negative events do occur in our lives, we are more likely to bounce back from them with ease and flow than someone who has not practiced Positive Psychology activities. We are more likely to accept that bad things happen to good people sometimes, and we are truly okay anyway. Our reactions to the event are less likely to be as dramatic as the event itself. We can live a fully engaged life sooner rather than later after the event.

My Story: change the language to change the mind

When my son Golden was a toddler, he was highly allergic to cats. We let him be around cats from time to time though, because the doctors felt that it would build his immunity and help him grow out of the allergy. They suggested we carry severe allergy eye drops when we visited people with cats, so we did.

One evening we went to dinner at a new church friend's apartment in downtown San Francisco. Cherry had a stunning, white, long-haired, Persian cat. My boy, being fascinated with its blue eyes and, long white fur, could not keep his hands off of Toby. After about fifteen minutes, Golden's eyes began to turn pink, and he started rubbing his itching, burning eyes. I looked through my "Mommy" bag, and to my utter disgust (and subsequent panic), I didn't have any eye drops. By this time Golden was in full blown tantrum mode, and rightly so.

I quickly gathered my things and my child, and we exited the apartment. In the lobby of the apartment building, I stopped for a few minutes. I sat down cross-legged and cradled him in my lap. I said softly, "Golden, close your eyes. Let's take the itch and pain away. Say *paining* with me. Let's say it over and over again."

Together, we repeated the word paining until it held no meaning. We turned the word pain (a noun) into an action word (a verb). We dove into the center of the word, the center of the meaning pain, until it disappeared. It dissipated into nothingness. Then the itchiness and burning disappeared as well. My toddler and I were able to finally get it together, exit the building, and go to a nearby drugstore to buy eye drops.

Positive Word Play

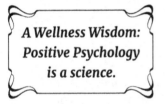

A Wellness Wisdom: Positive Psychology is a science.

I created this exercise in healing spontaneously, as I wanted to help my suffering son. I do not know where it came from, but my muse lives on my right shoulder.

I'm sharing this story because I see this word play as a sort of exercise in Positive Psychology. Golden had positive feelings after playing with the cat that surpassed the itchiness and burning. My son loved me unconditionally and trusted me to guide him through the word play. The word play was repetitive and a sort of meditative chant. We had practiced meditation throughout his babyhood, so it was familiar, like a mantra. He accepted the end result of getting to the center of the verb paining and the resulting end of pain. There was a positive spiral of events that led to the end of the itching and burning in a relatively short period of time. This all happened even before I could get him eye drops! We humans are powerful if we only have the belief that we are so. Positive word play can be a wellness tool to play around with.

I see negative reactions to negative events and painful emotions as verbs. Verbs are actions. It is my opinion that negative emotions and actions have an end point. Sooner or later they run out of gas. Just like the word pain, when I made it into paining and we repeated it, the word ran out of gas. Then we had a time of rest and relief.

Let's look at some examples of perceived negative action and emotion words:

- **hit=hitting**
  One will eventually tire of hitting and need to stop. The muscles will give out.

- **run=running**
  One will eventually have to stop running (or running away from problems, literally or figuratively) and rest, refuel, and rethink their situation.

- **hate=hating**
  One will eventually realize how exhausting hating is, and realize it is just an expression of fear turned inside out. Change the language, change the mindset.

- **eat=eating**
  Eating can only go on for so long until one gets sick and throws up. When eating is used in a negative and destructive manner, one will eventually stop, even if only for a little while before resuming the behavior. Stuffing emotions down with food is all too common in our society, but seeing it as a verb, an action word, may see an end to the action.

- **sleep=sleeping**
  Sleeping one's trouble's away doesn't work either. Eventually one will wake up to eat, use the restroom, go to work, or go to

school; perhaps someone who loves the distraught individual will intervene and get them out of bed.

No matter how expert the driver, the automobile will eventually run out of fuel in negativity, and the driver needs to accept that the vehicle needs a good dose of positive and restorative actions (gas or fuel).

An end to negativity is a beginning to positivity. Positive words seem to have no ending when made into a verb. Think of love.

- **love=loving**
  I see no end to loving. It doesn't tire me out. It generates energy rather than depleting it.

- **joy=joying**
  Is that even a word? (It is harder to make positive emotions into verbs for me.) Joy just *is*.

- **bliss=blissing**
  Get my point? Bliss just *is*.

Positive word play is a useful tool for one to engage in daily Positive Psychology. One of my yoga teachers had a great play on words that I want to share with you.

Ashleigh's Story: change=tranformation

Ashleigh is one of the yoga instructors at my local Bikram hot yoga studio. One day, when clearing out her dresser drawers, Ashleigh found a notebook from her teacher training days. She randomly flipped through the notebook and stumbled upon her own written words: **change=transformation**

In hot yoga, we let go of the pose held when the teacher says, "Change." During one afternoon class, Ashleigh said to the students, "What if every time we saw or thought the word *change,* we substituted the word *transform* for it?"

Wow. Just wow. Imagine the life we could have putting this into practice? Let's play with this concept:

- I'm going to change my clothes.=I'm going to transform my clothes.

- I'm going to change my bad habits.=I'm going to transform my bad habits.

- I'm going to change my life.=I'm going to transform my life.

- Do you need change for that?=Do you need transformation for that?

- Let me bring you the change.=Let me bring you transformation.

What a beautiful, uplifting life we can have just with a simple swap of words. I see this concept that Ashleigh suggested as a Positive Psychology tool in action. This can be applied all the time and everywhere. Plus, it is fun, humorous, whimsical, and free!

Gratitude: please and thank you go a long, long way

Practicing activities that show a big or small *thank you* is an expression of Positive Psychology. When we have an awareness of gratitude for the everyday little things, we are able to flourish as human beings and share more of who we are with the world. We seem to understand our purpose in the world. If we don't have a complete understanding, at least we are on our way. We are on the path with purpose. We are not lost.

I write down three things every evening that I am grateful for. Another thing I do that is a positive practice is collect fortunes from fortune cookies when I eat at Asian restaurants. I tape them in little notebooks with the date collected. When I hold the notebook in my hand, it gives me great pleasure and a surge of hope. I know they are manufactured in a mass way, without thought to who receives the fortune, but something magical seems possible every time I hold the notebook of fortunes!

An Invitation: gratitude letter

Write a meaningful letter by hand to a person who has had a beautiful and deep influence upon your life in a positive way. Tell them why, recalling as many details as possible. Either mail it to them or read it to them aloud in person. It will be a Positive Psychology activity for both of you and will be a moment neither of you will ever forget.

An Invitation: blessings

In a notebook, journal, or on a post-it pad, write down three things you were blessed with today. They may be large or small, significant or not. Make it a habit. Repetition is key in Positive Psychology. If the mind is resistant to change, it will begin to believe what was seemingly impossible only after consistent, repeated effort. One day, you will be surprised at your sunny outlook!

Positive Affirmations

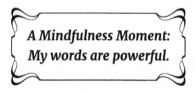

A Mindfulness Moment:
My words are powerful.

Positive affirmations are words and phrases we say aloud to ourselves several times a day that have a positive impact on our being. They are tools used in Positive Psychology (and in prayer rituals around the world). As we have learned earlier in this book, words are powerful. Let's take some time to love ourselves and choose words carefully to support who we truly are and who we truly want to be. An example of a positive affirmation may be as simple as, "I live life to the fullest." It may be a prayer or a song.

There are so many things out of our control on a daily basis. To bring a simple affirmation to one's life may be just the thing to effectively bring a sense of calm and control to the day. One can act and accomplish something that makes sense in a senseless world. We are addressing the daily stresses in a positive manner. There are even daily empowering quotes on smart phone apps these days (There's an app for that!). Taking the minute or two to read and reflect upon them is an exercise in Positive Psychology. It does a world of good, not only for you, but for the people whose lives you touch.

Positive affirmations are often statements of belief and intent. "I love myself completely. I am getting better in every way, every day." This is how we desire our lives to be. Through repetition, there is belief. Through belief, there is the creation of action in the body to support the belief. The more we use affirmations, the more our lives begin resembling them.

This is not just hippie-lovey-dovey talk. When we deliberately change our thoughts over a period of time, new neural pathways are formed in the brain to correspond with the new thoughts.[34] So, when a negative situation arises, the brain is not bound to automatically react to it in the way it used to. A new, more positive outcome is possible.

An Invitation: affirmation creation

Choose your own unique affirmation by thinking about what you want your new reality to be. Be positive and speak as if it is happening now. I call it the future-present. Say it or write it down fifteen times a day!

Examples:

- "I am healthy, wealthy, and wise."

- "I am at peace with the world and I love myself."

- "Money flows all around me. I'm prosperous and generous."

- "I radiate love and forgiveness."

- "My parenting skills are God based and loving."

- "I am not being judged by any other being. I am being loved by every other being."

Repetition is key. Feel free to add and drop affirmations when you feel it in your instincts, your soul spot. When one masters the life of one statement and owns it, there may be no use for the affirmation anymore. Release it. Make space, a sanctuary for a new one. Create or adopt another one.

To be completely honest, I feel like the previous chapters in this book are a collective testimony to Positive Psychology. I didn't have a label for it before, but the stories and exercises implemented throughout helped shape the lives of the affected persons for the better, long term. They healed through a variety of methods. Many rivers can lead to the sea of well being. Do I want one type of salad my whole life? Do I buy only apples at the fruit stand? No! Variety and experimentation is necessary to feel out what works for each individual person.

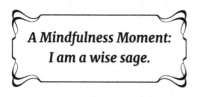

*A Mindfulness Moment:
I am a wise sage.*

We are different in our cultural backgrounds, our strengths, our levels of education, our chemical makeup, and what is considered acceptable to our belief systems. We wake up feeling different every day too, depending upon what we ate, drank, who we interacted with, and how we slept the night before. In order to get where we want to go in this life, we must take the first step. We take our glorious, beautiful, light-filled selves with us as we carry on through the daily tasks on earth, in this lifetime. Let's make the best of it, shall we?

Eat the rainbow of life and burst into a blooming *Happy, Healthy You.*

Chapter Seventeen

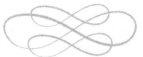

Gifts from My Elders ~ Being Open to Signs

My Uncle Joey grew to be a spiritual person later in his life, after his children were grown. Uncle Joey and I were close; he was my favorite uncle, and I was his favorite niece (I believe). We spoke of esoteric subjects privately, just between the two of us. About two weeks before his untimely death, he shared with me his wisdom of signs and symbolic messages in this world. We were talking by phone and he said to me, "Signs are everywhere. So many people are not open to signs, and then they are unaware of them. If people would be open to signs and invite them in, folks could receive them all day long, like mini-miracles. Imagine the sort of life you could have then, Kimmy."

He continued, "Then we have to know what to do with the signs we receive. We have to figure out the lesson or message and what to do with it."

I asked him if I could write about his wise advice in a blog or in my books, and he said, "Of course. Otherwise, why am I talking to you?"

Most people are too busy going through the tasks of everyday living. They are too busy or unwilling to let one more thing in, especially something that does not increase finances, conveniences, or creature comforts. I have always believed in signs, but Uncle Joey put the wisdom out there to me in a way that was easily understandable for all to receive.

To be aware of signs is tricky. For me, the first step is to invite symbols or signs into our lives. I do this by saying aloud or silently before I go to sleep, "Please send me a sign that teaches me a life lesson or allows me to do the same for others." I am open to receiving. With repetition of the invitation, the signs will eventually reveal themselves. Once that occurs over and over again, the awareness increases, and one can see signs and symbols with heavy meaning or affirmations. Sometimes they reveal themselves in quiet ways. Sometimes signs will reveal themselves through dreams. I know. Or, I believe I know. And why not? I am deserving. So are you.

Signs from Dreams

My most recent signs have come to me in dreams. Recently I listened to a podcast by a PhD in psychology, and he said the answers to his deeper questions came from God, Spirit, or his muse. Unfortunately they woke him up at 3:13 a.m. Then he had to write the information down immediately to help his clients, his writing, his patients, or with his personal questions. I heard that part of the interview and just shook my head because I was not open to that time frame. I love to sleep 9-10 hours a night.

Wouldn't you know it, my muse had other ideas? I dreamed I was in a Ross Dress for Less store, looking at change purses and wallets in the accessory area. I kept finding wads of money and lots of coins with notes written on the leather interior or cloth interior from a woman named Sarah. She wrote inside the wallets and coin purses that if I found this, then I must really need the money and the encouragement that I was worthy. I must do something good for my family and friends with the money, and use my newfound money for good. Enhancing my life through my own good fortune and passing it on was the lesson for me in the sign. When I woke up from the dream it was 4:29 a.m. I repeated the dream over and over again softly so I wouldn't forget it. Plus, I was too lazy to get up and write it down with pen and paper.

The second dream that night with signs was just as prolific for me. I was reading college textbooks on the history of the world as well as US history. I was repeating and repeating the dates and facts as I was rushing to the university to take tests. I remember catching up with a history professor and yelling at him, "Why are we memorizing and memorizing? It serves no one in our modern times unless I relate facts and dates to what I do in my daily world now! It helps me not one bit unless it creates in me a kinder, gentler, and more compassionate human experience. We students seek connection, relationships, and our goal as humans is to spread love above all!"

The professor stopped in his tracks and smiled widely at me. "Well, we traditional educators never thought of history in that way before. Wow. You have got something special there!" I woke up from that dream at 5:27 a.m. I was still too lazy to get up and write it down.

How do these signs from my dreams talk to me and teach me something? Do they teach me something I can share with you? The first dream has become the basis of my holiday gift giving. I go to stores all season long to place coins in small envelopes and quietly stuff them anonymously in wallets and change purses with notes of guidance to do *good* with the money. What a personal revelation. I invite you to do the same. It can be our own Secret Santa project, all around the world.

The second dream contained signs and symbols which taught me that whatever mundane tasks we must do just to get through to the end of the day, the end of the season, the end of the semester, etc., can be for good. We can spread love and connection through the murkiness of memorizing what we think of as boring. Use the knowledge, the tests, the patience earned with limitations and confrontations as a way to *see,* really *see* the big picture. What are we doing this stuff for? Just to say we did it, we got through it? No, we finish the task to say we did it in a way that becomes a vehicle for higher elevation and love in all facets of our lives.

A Wellness Wisdom:
Be open to receiving
new information in
unusual ways, and
then open to sharing
it with others who
are trusting in your
intentions.

I know driving to work every day sucks, but what if one day on the commute, you listened to a mind blowing podcast or radio show that changes the way you forever answer the question, "How are you?" How many times a day do we ask and hear that question?

Invite the signs, receive the signs, be aware that they are signs, interpret the signs, and act upon the signs in your own unique way.

My Story: walk and don't walk signs

I was walking to work in downtown San Francisco, when I looked across the street at the crosswalk sign. A man, dressed in khaki pants and a polo shirt was performing pull-ups by jumping up and grabbing the metal poles where the "walk" and "don't walk" lights were placed. I was amazed at his tenacity and discipline to do what he needed to do in order to meet his life goals, which obviously included improving or practicing his physical strength. I was so impressed. Maybe some folks thought he was crazy or homeless. To me, it was a sign given to me by the Universe, God, my guides, or whatever you want to call it. I observed a real-life example of a thought that has not left my head for weeks: "Allow no one to steal your joy."

I do not think the example was given to me by accident. I was given a sign that day, and through time and repetition, I have learned to be aware of signs. I then could use it for my own growth, and use the lesson for sharing here and now. I believe the Universe placed a concrete example in my path in order to further explain to you the meaning of allowing no one to steal your goals or your joy.

Past Life Cynicism

Like many of you, I need proof of things. We live in a science-driven, data-driven society nowadays. I want a receipt when I buy groceries or clothes to prove that I purchased the items, or in case I want to return them. The subject of reincarnation has fascinated me for years, and many people have sworn they know who they were before or had a hypnotist help them meditate to find deeper meaning to this life through a past life regression meditation. I myself participated in a past life regression course when I was in my thirties. I was keenly interested in anything esoteric or metaphysical at that time. I was cynical then because of the lack of proof, but hopeful because I wanted to know myself better.

I remember quietly lying down in a room with about thirty other people. The psychologist hosting the workshop took us on a guided, closed eye meditation, a journey of sorts to our own past lives. After we were aroused from the meditation we shared our experiences.

I discovered that I was an African American, male piano player in the late 1930's. I had a female fiancée who was also my singer/ partner. We were a duo who performed in little ragtime clubs somewhere in the deep southern states of the USA. I remembered my personal motto: *A little ditty and a smile will make your day.* I remembered my linen pants, my fancy shoes, and my leather briefcase stuffed with piano sheet music. I remembered my light, caramel colored hands, with the veins bulging as my fingers flew across the keys. My sweetie and I were to be married soon, but unfortunately I was drafted into the armed services.

I was not a fighter by nature, and I was an untalented soldier. A few months into my active duty during World War II, I was killed on a battlefield. While I was dying, I remembered regretting not being able to marry and live a long time with the love of my life.

When we came out of the regression meditation, the psychologist asked the participants to share what we learned from the past life experience. I said that my message from my past was to live *this* life without regrets. I then asked the psychologist, "What if I made this all up? What if it was just my imagination?" The reply was that if it taught me *anything* about myself, then that was the meaningful purpose of the exercise.

<hr />

I See Miracles Every Day Now

As of this writing in 2017, finally California is officially out of the drought. It has been raining for a few months almost every day, a normal rainy season. One Monday night when it was raining and hailing, Sage, my twelve-year old daughter, and I were walking across the street in a cross walk that was clearly marked. All of the cars in both directions had stopped. It was a residential district except for an organic deli on one corner. The speed limit was 25 miles per hour. Out of nowhere, a woman in a silver sedan veered around all of the stopped cars in the cross walk, driving way past the speed limit and almost hit Sage. I grabbed Sage by her shoulder and pulled her back toward me just in the nick of time. It was literally less than an inch between life and death.

The woman was on a giant white phone held up to her ear. She did not stop. I saw that she had zero expression on her face. When

Sage and I got to the other side of the street to the sidewalk, I pulled her to me closely. I put my hands around her face and said, "Do you realize what just happened?" She nodded yes. I repeated myself and she nodded again. I started spouting off things like, "What if she had hit you? What if Golden was an only child again? You are my baby, my only daughter. You could have been killed by a woman who was simply distracted."

I further explained that the woman was probably not a jerk. She was probably a good hearted human being. What if she was having her own family emergency right then and there and she was on her way home to handle it? I encouraged Sage to be mindful and present every time she crossed the street and especially when she began driving in a few years.

As we drove home, I began to get more emotional: I teared up and felt nauseous. Sage was quiet. "I think I'm going to be sick." I opened my car door and puked at a stop sign twice on the way home. When we arrived home I called Golden into the kitchen. After he heard my tone of voice, "Get in the kitchen, right now…" he knew something important was up. As I relayed the story, Golden put his arms around Sage and me, and our three foreheads touched. We were in a circle of thanks, realizing the miracle that had just occurred. Golden got teary-eyed, and seeing this from her big brother, Sage was able to finally release too. Of course I had been crying non-stop since she was almost hit.

I'm telling you this story because ever since that miraculous evening, guests at the restaurant where I work have been openly telling me their miracles, their deepest life stories, whether I share anything about that rainy evening or not. It is as if my unspoken energy invites them to share their journeys with me. And, without me saying a word, they are telling me to share…Now that is what I call complete encouragement and a definite sign from the Universe that I am becoming a *Happy, Healthy Me.*

Soon after the miracle of Sage not being hit by the car, a group of three guests, a man and two women, came into my restaurant and were seated at one of my tables. They were chatting and having a great time, and enjoying my entertaining service as well. At the end of the meal, they had a lot of leftovers which I offered to box up for them. They said they were in San Francisco for the fancy food show and snacked all day as part of their duties, so they didn't need leftovers for snacks.

I told them one my favorite satiating snacks to keep in my car were peanuts with the shells on, raw or roasted, because of the fiber, fat, and protein they contain. I went on and on, probably because I had no other tables left and I had consumed a lot of coffee that evening. I talked about fiber and the many uses of peanut fiber and the science of nuts in general. They started laughing and said, "Do you know what we do?" I said, "No." The gentleman at the table said, "The two ladies across from me are food scientists and we are here at the fancy food show representing the largest peanut company in the world. We distribute peanuts to Planters, to Godiva chocolates, to See's candies, to Snickers, to grocery store brands, as dollar store off-brand peanuts in a bag, shell on, shell off, almost every peanut food you can think of has our peanuts in them."

How amazing that they sat at my table when the restaurant was nearing closing time and they had the choice of any table in the room. I pushed the envelope a little. I continued to ask them if they believed in signs. The gentleman said definitely yes. The ladies agreed. Before they left, I asked them the name of their company. The name of their company is Golden Peanut Company. I smiled widely and quietly stated, "Now if that's not a sign that you were meant to be in my space tonight, I don't know what is. My first born is named Golden." We all embraced as they left the restaurant.

Jolly Ramblings

I met a new coworker for the first time the other day and his name was Jolly. He said his brother was named Lucky. I asked him if he had good days every day due to his name. He smiled at me and replied, "Most days I live up to my name." That got me thinking about names. What if you could choose your name and express with your name who you feel you are inside at your core? I know two friends who have done a legal name change, and they are so joyful about it.

Once we heal from unfortunate situations we may have some wonderful self discoveries. We may be more open to others than before. We may be spontaneous for the first time ever. We may trust our instincts more easily. We may build a tribe of close friends who are like minded. We may try new activities and engage in personal development with fervor. We may just be a bit more content, with a little smile under the surface rather than a scowl most of the day. Here are some ideas that popped into my head once I got the monkey off my back:

- What about a free pass day? If you had no responsibilities for a day, what would your perfect day look like? Be creative. Jot down ideas and perhaps turn the plan into action.

- Have you ever wanted an un-wedding? So many folks are happy being single or attached without a legal document, but they know exactly where they would want a wedding party. They fantasize about the food and the décor. Why wait? Have an un-wedding.

- My cousin Annie and I used to live together in Los Angeles. Every month we had theme parties with our tribe of close support. Everyone would bring a dish, keeping it an economical way for us to gather and connect with those who meant the most to us. February was heart-shaped food month,

March was green food month, April was water-filled fruits and veggies or rainy day movies and popcorn, etc.

There are no holes in your soul, my friends. I learned that through my life experiences just as you are learning. We are encouraged to reduce, reuse, and recycle material things. What if we did that with our troubles and worries? Live more simply by reducing the difficult situations to the smallest denominator by using the invitations throughout this book. Reuse the activities that give you the biggest return on happy feelings. Recycle means to convert waste into a reusable material. I encourage you to convert your troubles into something creative. Use the energy in a new way.

There are no holes in your soul, just like there are no holes in the car when I can't find something that I dropped while driving. I just have to pull over, take my time, and put an effort into finding the item, like a good detective. Let's be a detective for ourselves, and work towards looking out for our higher happiness. I invite you to be a sleuth for a *Happy, Healthy You.*

Conclusion

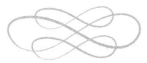

There are some people who can't seem to get out of their own way. I'm one of those people. You are too. Some of the time, we all wear that hat, and we seem like buffoons to ourselves and to everybody around us. Our self destructive patterns may not be obvious or grand, but they are there, slightly under the surface, like the person who knows how to straighten up the house when Mom comes to visit, but all the crap is swept under the rug until she leaves (college, anyone?); it hurts a little bit to admit this, especially since we all appear so polished on the outside. "Aaaaagh, why did I do this $#!+ again?" Stop the sense of devaluation of the self – let go of the ego, right now.

To truly transform ourselves takes some *aha* moments, as mentioned numerous times throughout this book. When we experience such an epiphany, we can live in a way that hits all of our cylinders, not just a few of them. We can learn what our spiritual perspectives are, too. Then we must make our goals apparent to ourselves, create an action plan, and confirm our commitment to effort. I call these the Three D's. The Three D's are **DESIRE, DETERMINATION, AND DEDICATION.**

- Desire

- Determination

- Dedication

These D words have morphed over the years to become my family mantra. They hold great meaning for my family in spelling out how to find recovery and healing from life's many crises, as well as assisting in my personal life goals. This is a powerful technique in the total wellness toolkit.

- **Desire** is the end result, the goal that one wants. State it and write it down. Say it loud and say it proud! This is your future calling!

- **Determination** is the process that one goes through in order to make that happen. Once the steps are revealed as to what to do (the exercises in this book), stick to it and follow the steps in order.

- **Dedication** is the commitment one has to seeing the whole thing through to the finish line.

Together, these Three D's spell out personal victory over the demons and the distractions. The Three D's can be used for reaching, and then facing your superior self. Challenge yourself with new health, mind, heart, and spiritual wellness quests. Follow the Three D's by writing it all down in that little notebook, and then GO! When we utilize the Three D's, we can trigger a lot of different healthier choices and we will see positive patterns emerge.

In my opinion, the Three D's method is an approachable and attainable method of healing, if we stop acting out of self-hate. When I help others who want to take the Three D's approach, I help people discover how they got into the state of self-doubt and self-loathing. Then we find out how they used certain patterns and habits to confirm the negative self-beliefs.

When we dedicate ourselves to better health, we are supporting and boosting all of the relationships and facets of our lives. We are integrated beings, after all. Therefore, we must work on all levels, mind, body, and spirit. Wake up! It's time for a brand new internal dialogue and way of living that nurtures us into becoming a different sort of human being. I believe in you, so YOU believe in you too.

I know that wellness can be many things to many people. It can be inside of us and outside of us. Our minds, bodies, and spirits deserve to be in balance. When we reach that place, we can operate optimally and feel healthy and whole again. Can we expand beyond what we see right now? In every aspect of our lives, we can back up and away a little in order to see the big picture. Then we can keep moving the line of limitation, one millimeter at a time, until we feel limitless in our possibilities.

As I stated earlier in this book, my journey to wellness began with food. When I feed my body with nutrient dense, life and energy giving foods, my cells are being well fed at their very center. That in turn converts into brain and body power that I feel from my head to my toes. I believe I have become more loving, more intelligent, and more spiritual since changing my eating template to whole, real foods. I swear, I sometimes physically sense the moment that my body begins absorbing all the goodness! There is an internal humming, a buzzing, a *zing* I sense. Soon after eating, I feel stronger and smarter, and sometimes I burst into laughter, song, or explode with creative thoughts! I invite you to feel the same things.

So the question is now, can we persist in the face of life's struggles? Are we able to reclaim the glorious life? Do we want it bad enough to do the work and soul searching? Can we get uncomfortable in order to finally be comfortable?

Life is like a grocery run for me now. I know I need something. I'm empty. So I get in the car, fasten my seat belt, and go on a road trip. When I get to the store, I never know what I'm going to pick up, but I know my foundation, my staples. Our healing and growing from our mistakes and troubles are like the grocery run too.

There is no time limit to healing. I compare the time it takes to recover, heal, and spring forth to making fermented vegetables. When I make sauerkraut or pickled vegetables, it takes time.

Sometimes it ferments in a week. Sometimes it takes a month or more to ferment properly and for the flavor profiles and good probiotics to transform the salt, brine, and veggies into health giving, immune building foods. Each strain of good bacteria is like replanting a beautiful variety of flower species in the garden, that is, the intestines. When done well, the garden grows and also protects the environment. And so it is with our mental strength and clarity. We don't *get it* until we do. That's why there are so many types of exercises here. You never know which one will resonate with you until you do them. You cannot speed up understanding…

Yes, healing from being incredibly broken takes long-term effort. It's not easy or sexy to fix long-term suffering. Heavy challenges usually cannot be fixed with short-term answers. If short cuts are the normal way, then failure results again and again. With long-term commitment, we *will* get to the happy ending, and the satisfaction *will* show us how worthwhile it was to stay on track. Life happens. When we are physically and mentally armed with the tools and resources here, we can thrive (rather than survive) during hard times. Stuff comes up. It is imperative to go for it and rise above these challenges. In the end, we will be uplifted, instead of staying stuck in a dark place just going through the motions to survive. We do have the ability to live a fully engaged life.

Every day, every week, every month, and every year, we will face life moments that aren't *normal*. There are many ways to lose the baggage and blame, once and for all. I wanted to pass on to you what I have learned about changing the way I eat, play, think, and love. I eat, play, think, and love so that I can attain and maintain healthy moods when life challenges occur. With this knowledge comes the responsibility to share my findings, which have been truly life-changing for me, and for the people who I help daily.

I believe we should embrace our emotions, not deny them. Emotions = energy + motion. That is, they are our strong feelings, which are backed by energy, moving through us. If the energy is backed up and it doesn't flow properly, we can shatter like a cold glass when hot water is poured into it. (That's a mess I don't want or need to clean up!) We can work with and through our emotions, and see how they may better serve us and our higher purpose. We do have the strength (even if it's hard to believe) to forge ahead and attempt our best life, even if our lives are pretty spectacular already. I want us to sit in the seat of hope and fasten our seat belts tightly. Then it's take-off time! It's time to work diligently towards becoming our most authentic self, our superior self.

Even when there is a positive resolution to the crappy events that have held us back before, that doesn't mean other struggles won't present themselves in the future. Now, however, we are more armed and ready, after working with the exercises in this book. The multidisciplinary approach within these pages will help you get unstuck, and then a natural flow of action will be available to you when the challenges arise. What can our human potential do with that?

"The ultimate lesson all of us have to learn is unconditional love, which includes not only others but ourselves as well."
—Elisabeth Kubler-Ross, psychiatrist, author

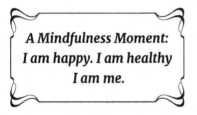

A Mindfulness Moment:
I am happy. I am healthy
I am me.

I don't have a better answer for you than this book. I have spent years searching for answers, researching, experimenting, and then sharing the results, so that you may fly. I truly do not want to be *normal* or *invisible*. Do you? It is time to shed self-blame, lose the baggage, trauma, and drama. Meet your *Happy, Healthy You.*

Bibliography

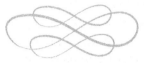

Adams, Mike. *Extreme Health Radio Podcast*. Episode 298, August 13, 2014.

Asprey, Dave, and Asprey, Lana, M.D. *The Better Baby Book*. Hoboken, New Jersey: John Wiley and Sons, Inc., 2013.

Bach, Richard. *Running from Safety*. Rockland, Maryland: Wheeler Publishing, Inc., 1994.

Baker, Dan, PhD, and Greenberg, Cathy, PhD. with Yalof, Ina. *What Happy Women Know: How New Findings in Positive Psychology Can Change Women's Lives for the Better*. New York: Rodale Press, 2007.

Bart, Teddy, and Evins, Karlen. *Beyond Reason Podcast. http://www.beyondreason.com*

Benoit, Michael. *Giving Psychology Away Podcast*. Self Control, Self Discipline, and Positive Psychology, Episode 3, February 28, 2007.

Berkson, D. Lindsey. *Hormone Deception*. Chicago: Contemporary Books, 2000.

Bhaerman, Steve, and Lipton, Bruce H., Ph.D. *Spontaneous Evolution: Our Positive Future*. Carlsbad, California: Hay House, 2009.

Bogart, Greg. *Meditation and Psychotherapy, American Journal of Psychotherapy*,110-113, 1991.

Broad, William. *The Science of Yoga: The Risks and the Rewards*. New York: Simon and Schuster, 2012.

Campbell-McBride, Natasha, MD. *Gut and Psychology Syndrome.* Cambridge, UK: Medinform Publishing, 2010.

Carey, Nessa. *The Epigenetics Revolution.* New York: Columbia University Press, 2012.

Carper, Cara, and Kvist, Darlene, CNS. *Dishing Up Nutrition Podcast.* Food, Brain Chemistry, and Eating Disorders, Interview with Lea Wetzell and Jennifer Schmid, Episode November 30, 2014. *http://weightandwellness.com*

Chaney, Michael, Haugon, David M., and Musser, Susan. *Depression.* Farmington Hills, Michigan: Greenhaven Press, 2014.

Chase, Richard B., PhD, and Dasu, Sriram, PhD. *The Customer Service Solution.* New York: McGraw Hill Education, 2013.

Choudry, Bikram. *Bikram Yoga.* New York: Harper Collins, 2007.

Claire, Robin. *Tributaries Radio Podcast.*

Coleman, Lee H., PhD, ABPP. *Depression: A Guide for the Newly Diagnosed.* Oakland, California: New Harbinger Publications, Inc., 2012.

Cook, Mary Lou, Fisher, Diane, and Frigo, Victoria. *You Can Help Someone Who is Grieving.* New York: Penguin, 1996.

Cope, Andy, and Whittaker, Andy. *Be Brilliant Every Day.* West Sussex, UK: Capstone, 2012.

Crapo, Lawrence. *Hormones: The Messengers of Life.* New York: W.H. Freeman and Company, 1985.

Dr. Pieter DeWet Live Podcast. Women's Health, Hahimoto's Disease and Hypothyroidism, Episode May 15, 2014.

Elliot, Charles H., PhD, and Smith, Laura L., PhD. *Depression for Dummies.* Indianapolis, Indiana: Wiley Publishing, Inc., 2003.

Ellsworth, Abigail, and Altman, Peggy. *Massage Anatomy.* San Diego, CA: Thunder Bay Press, 2009.

Feldman, David B., PhD, and Kravetz, Lee Daniel. *Supersurvivors: The Surprising Link Between Suffering and Success.* New York: Harper Wave, 2014.

Finkelhor, D., & Browne, A. *The Traumatic Impact of Child Sexual Abuse: A Conceptualization. American Journal of Orthopsychiatry*, 55, 530-541, 1985.

Finley, Guy. *The Courage to Be Free*. San Francisco: Red Wheel/Weiser Books, 2010.

Finley, Guy. *Let Go and Live in the Now*. Boston: Red Wheel/Weiser Books, 2004.

Fox, Elaine. *Rainy Brain, Sunny Brain*. New York: Basic Books, 2012.

Francis, Richard C. *Epigenetics: The Ultimate Mystery of Inheritance*. New York: W.W. Norton & Co., 2011.

Fried, George H., PhD, and Hademenos, George J., PhD. *Biology*. New York: McGraw Hill, 2013.

Goode, Julie-Anne, M.A., MFT1. *Psych 1 On 1 Podcast*. Somatic Therapy, The Mind-Body Connection Episode, December 5, 2015.

Gottfried, Sara, MD. *The Hormone Cure*. New York: Scribner, 2013.

Gray, Tyrus. *The End Depression Podcast*. Episode 1, December 9, 2012.

Guenther, Ernest. *The Essential Oils, Vol. 1*. New York: Fritzsche Brothers, Inc., 1947.

Hanson, Rick, Ph.D. *Hardwiring Happiness*. New York: Harmony Books, 2013.

Hazelton, Suzanne. *Great Days at Work: How Positive Psychology Can Transform Your Working Life*. London: Kogan Page, 2013.

Herman, Judith, M.D. *Trauma and Recovery*. New York: Basic Books, 1997.

James, Sophie, and Lee, Deborah A. *The Compassionate-Mind Guide to Recovering from Trauma and PTSD*. Oakland, California: New Harbinger Publications, 2011.

Kessler, David, and Kubler-Ross, Elisabeth, M.D. *Life Lessons:Two Experts on Death and Dying Teach Us the Mysteries of Life and Living*. New York: Scribner, 2000.

Kubler-Ross, Elisabeth, M.D. *On Death and Dying: What the Dying Have to Teach Doctors, Nurses, Clergy, and Their Own Families.* New York: Scribner, 1969.

Kushner, Harold. *When Bad Things Happen to Good People.* New York: Schocken Books, 1981.

Laake, Dana, and Passero, Dr. Kevin. *Essentials of Healthy Living Podcast.*

Landis, KJ. *Superior Self: Reaching Superior Health For A Superior Self.* Bloomington, Indiana: Balboa Press, 2014.

LaRoche, Loretta. *Relax---You May Only Have a Few Minutes Left.* Carlsbad, California: Hay House Inc., 2008.

Leimbach, Claire, and McShane, Trypheyna. *The Intimacy of Death and Dying.* Crows Nest, NSW, Australia: Allen and Unwin, 2009.

Levenkron, Steven. *Stolen Tomorrows: Understanding and Treating Women's Childhood Sexual Abuse.* New York: W.W. Norton & Co., Inc., 2007.

Levine, Stephen. *Unattended Tomorrow: Recovering from Loss and Reviving the Heart.* Emmaus, Pennsylvania: Rodale, Inc., 2005.

Lubarsky, Alex. *Health Media Podcast. http://www.navelexpo.com*

Lustig, Robert, M.D. *Fat Chance: Beating the Odds Against Sugar, Processed Food, Obesity, and Disease.* NewYork: Hudson Street Press, 2013.

Maccaro, Janet, PhD, CNC. *Change Your Food, Change Your Mood.* Lake Mary, Florida: Siloam, A Strang Company, 2008.

Marsico, Katie. *Depression and Stress.* New York: Cavendish Square Publishing, 2014.

Martinez, Mario Dr. *The Mind Body Code.* Boulder, Colorado: Sounds True, 2014.

McKenna, Paul, PhD. *Change Your life in 7 Days.* New York: Sterling, 2010.

McNaughton, Ian. *Body, Breath, Consciousness*. Berkeley, California: North Atlantic Books, 2004.

Noonan, Susan J., M.D., M.P.H. *Managing Your Depression:What You Can Do to Feel Better*. Baltimore: The Johns Hopkins University Press, 2013.

O'Connor, Richard, PhD. *Rewire: Change Your Brain to Break Bad Habits, Overcome Addictions, & Conquer Self-Destructive Behavior*. New York: Hudson Street Press, 2014.

Parry, Vivienne. *The Truth About Hormones*. London: Atlantic Books, 2005.

Perlmutter, David, MD. with Loberg, Kristen. *Brain Maker*. New York: Little, Brown & Company, 2015.

Peterson, Christopher. *A Primer in Positive Psychology*. New York: Oxford University Press, 2006.

Podder, Tanushree. *The Magic of Massage*. New Delhi: V & S Publishers, 2011.

Rawlings, Deidre, Ph.D., N.D. Fermented Foods for *Health*. Beverly, Massachusetts: Fair Winds Press, 2013.

Reinagel, Monica with guest Hendriksen, Ellen, M.D. *The Nutrition Diva's Quick and Dirty Tips for Eating Well and Feeling Fabulous Podcast*. Episode 283, How Food Affects Mood, May 13, 2014. *http://www.quickanddirtytips.com*

Ross, Julia. *The Mood Cure: The Four Step Program to Rebalance Your Emotional Chemistry and Rediscover Your Natural Sense of Well Being*. New York: Viking, 2002.

Schiraldi, Glen, Ph.D. *The Post-Traumatic Stress Disorder Sourcebook*. New York:McGraw Hill, 2009.

Seligman, Martin, Ph. D. *Authentic Happiness*. New York: Atria, 2002.

Singh, Simran. *11:11 Talk Radio Podcast*.

Souza Ma, Christina. *Trinity of Life Podcast. http://www.yogahub. tv*

Strauss, Abby. *Florida Psychiatric Society Podcast*. Interview with Garrie Thompson and Norman Fine on Surviving After a Loved One's Suicide, Episode from November 7, 2010. *http://wwww.afsp.org*

Strozzi-Heckler, Richard. *The Art of Somatic Coaching*. Berkeley, California: North Atlantic Books, 2014.

Tindle, Hilary, M.D., M.P.H. *Up: How Positive Outlook Can Transform Our Health and Aging*. New York: Hudson Street Press, 2013.

Trappler, Brian, M.D. *Identifying and Recovering from Psychological Trauma*. New York: Gordian Knot Books, 2009.

Treumpy, Kristen. *The Positive Psychology Podcast*. Strengths, Episode 2, August 23, 2014.

Walker, Pete. *Complex PTSD: From Surviving to Thriving*. Lafayette, California: Azure Coyote Book, 2014.

Walsh, William J., PhD. *Nutrient Power: Heal Your Biochemistry and Heal Your Brain*. New York: Skyhorse Publishing, 2014.

Welch, Claudia Dr., MSOM. *Balance Your Hormones, Balance Your Life*. Philadelphia, Pennsylvania: DaCapo Press, 2011.

Worwood, Valerie Ann. *The Complete Book of Essential Oils and Aromatherapy*. Novato, CA: New World Library, 2016.

Websites

http://wwww.afsp.org

http://arthritis.org

http://laughteryoga.org

http://lindencenterofhope.org

http://www.medicinenet.com

http://myvillagegreen.com

http://www.navelexpo.com

http://www.quickanddirtytips.com

http://weightandwellness.com

http://www.yogahub.tv

About the Author

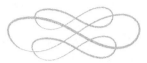

KJ Landis is an author, educator and health and life coach. She holds a Bachelor of Science in Education, and has certificates in Personal Training, Fitness Class Instructing, as well as certificates in continuing education in Psychology, Global Health, Childhood Development and Nutrition at Stanford School of Medicine, Johns Hopkins University, and other prestigious universities.

Her focus is on teaching restorative practices for healing, a grain free and sugar free lifestyle, and how to build a tribe of support when making any lifestyle change for the better. Landis consults clients locally in San Francisco and remotely via internet and phone. She creates and facilitates wellness workshops in libraries, senior centers, corporations, and private homes.

KJ Landis has been a featured guest on numerous podcasts and is an in-demand motivational speaker. She has written numerous books on wellness. Her weekly videos and blogs share holistic health topics as well as provide motivational and inspirational support. KJ is the founder and CEO of Superior Self®. She is the creator of Superior Self's Guide to Wellness from Within and the Eat Well, Be Well 30 Day Transformation Program. You may read more about KJ Landis and her personal journey to wellness at www.superiorselfwithkjlandis.com.

Her ability to communicate effectively, compassionately, and with patience has helped build self-esteem and attainment of others' life goals.

Currently KJ Landis lives and works in San Francisco. She has a husband and two children.

End Notes

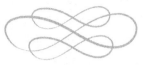

1. My husband has many one liners that are profound statements for me. This quote came from him, Torino Von Jones

2. KJ Landis, *Superior Self: Reaching Superior Health For A Superior Self* (Bloomington, IN: Balboa Press, 2014).

3. Landis, *Superior Self: Reaching Superior Health For A Superior Self*, Chapter 5.

4. Natasha Campbell-McBride, M.D., *Gut and Psychology Syndrome* (Cambridge, UK: Medinform Publishing, 2010).

5. Brian Trappler, M.D., *Identifying and Recovering from Psychological Trauma* (New York: Gordian Knot Books, 2009).

6. Trappler, M.D., *Identifying and Recovering from Psychological Trauma*.

7. Steven Levenkron, *Stolen Tomorrows: Understanding and Treating Women's Childhood Sexual Abuse* (New York: W.W. Norton and Company, 2007).

8. http:/www.laughteryoga.org

9. http:/www.arthritis.org

10. Stephen Levine, *Unattended Tomorrow: Recovering from Loss and Reviving the Heart* (Emmaus, PA: Rodale Inc, 2005).

11. Elisabeth Kubler-Ross, M.D., *On Death and Dying: What the Dying Have to Teach Doctors, Nurses, Clergy, and Their Own Families* (New York: Scribner, 1969).

12. Bum Jin Park, Yuko Tsunetsugu, and Yoshifumi Miyazaki, *The Physiological Effects of Shinrin-yoku: Evidence from Field Experiments in 24 Forests Across Japan, Environmental Health and Preventive Medicine* (2010; 15 (1): 18-26), http:/www.ncbi.nim.gov/pmc/articles/PMC27933.

13. http:/www.shinrin-yoku.org

14. Bruce H. Lipton, PhD., and Steve Bhaerman, *Spontaneous Evolution: Our Positive Future* (Carlsbad, CA: Hay House, 2009).

15. Nessa Carey, *The Epigenetics Revolution* (New York: Columbia University Press, 2012).

16. Nessa Carey, *The Epigenetics Revolution.*

17. Nessa Carey, *The Epigenetics Revolution.*

18. Lee H. Coleman, PhD., *Depression: A Guide for the Newly Diagnosed* (Oakland, CA: New Harbinger Publications, 2012).

19. http:/www.ncbi.nim.gov/pmc/articles/PMC27933.

20. William T. Walsh, PhD., *Nutrient Power: Heal Your Biochemistry and Heal Your Brain* (New York: Skyhorse Publishing, 2014).

21. Dr. Ellen Hendriksen, guest of Monica Reinagel, *The Nutrition Diva's Quick and Dirty Tips for Eating Well and feeling Fabulous Podcast* (Episode 283, May 13, 2014, "How Food Affects Mood"). http:/www.quickanddirtytips.com.

22. Susan J. Noonan, M.D., PhD., *Managing Your Depression: What You Can Do to Feel Better* (Baltimore, MD: The Johns Hopkins University Press, 2013)

23. Chris Randall, *"Measuring National Well Being: Our Relationships, 2015,"* (UK: Office for National Statistics, 2015). http:/www.ons.gov.uk.

24. Vivienne Parry, *The Truth About Hormones* (London: Atlantic Books, 2005).

25. Vivienne Parry, *The Truth About Hormones*.

26. Janet Maccaro, PhD., *Change Your Food, Change Your Mood* (Lake Mary, FL.: Siloam, A Strang Company, 2008).

27. Karen J. Miller, PhD., and Steven A. Rogers, PhD., *The Estrogen-Depression Connection* (Oakland, CA: New Harbinger Publications, 2007).

28. Richard Strozzi-Heckler, *The Art of Somatic Coaching* (Berkeley, CA: North Atlantic Books, 2014).

29. Dr. Mario Martinez, *The Mind-Body Code* (Boulder, CO: Sounds True, 2014).

30. Dr. Mario Martinez, *The Mind-Body Code*.

31. Christopher Peterson, *A Primer in Positive Psychology* (New York: Oxford University Press, 2006).

32. Hilary Tindle, M.D., M.P.H., *Up: How Positive Outlook Can Transform Our Health and Aging* (New York:Hudson Street Press, 2013).

33. Dan Baker, PhD., and Cathy Greenberg, PhD., *What Happy Women Know: How New findings in Positive Psychology Can Change Women's Lives for the Better* (Emmaus, PA: Rodale Press, 2007).

34. Rick Hanson, PhD., *Hardwiring Happiness* (New York: Harmony Books, 2013).

CPSIA information can be obtained
at www.ICGtesting.com
Printed in the USA
BVOW09s1505080817
491440BV00001B/1/P